# MCQs for FRCOphth and ICO Basic Sciences Examinations

## SAMEER TRIKHA
BM BSc (Hons) MRCOphth
Specialty Registrar, Ophthalmology
Southampton General Hospital, Southampton, UK

## SAMANTHA DE SILVA
MA MRCP MRCOphth
Specialty Registrar, Ophthalmology
John Radcliffe Hospital, Oxford, UK

## HEMAL MEHTA
MA MBBS
Specialty Registrar, Ophthalmology
Moorfields Eye Hospital, London, UK

## SIMON KEIGHTLEY
FRCS FRCOphth
Consultant Ophthalmic Surgeon
North Hampshire Hospital, Basingstoke, UK

*Foreword by*
**ANDREW LOTERY**
MD FRCOphth
Professor of Ophthalmology
Southampton General Hospital, UK

**CRC Press**
Taylor & Francis Group
Boca Raton London New York

CRC Press is an imprint of the
Taylor & Francis Group, an **informa** business

**Radcliffe Publishing Ltd**
33–41 Dallington Street
London
EC1V 0BB
United Kingdom

www.radcliffepublishing.com

British Library Cataloguing in Publication Data

A catalogue record for this book is available from the British Library.

ISBN-13: 978 184619 546 4

The paper used for the text pages of this book
is FSC® certified. FSC (The Forest Stewardship
Council®) is an international network to promote
responsible management of the world's forests.

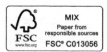

Typeset by Darkriver Design, Auckland, New Zealand

# Contents

# Foreword

It is refreshing to see a new comprehensive question book to assist candidates undertaking the FRCOphth and ICO Basic Science exams. This up-to-date book will give candidates much-needed practice with the type of questions that they are likely to encounter in these examinations. Thus, it should significantly increase their chances of success.

The authors have considerable experience of these types of examinations, both as trainees and examiners. As a result, they have produced detailed and comprehensive coverage of the curriculum. The material is clearly organised by topic, allowing ease of revision. The book has a clear style and, unusually for this type of book, also provides detailed and well-explained answers. I am sure it will have wide appeal both to exam candidates and also to ophthal-mologists seeking to refresh their knowledge or undertake revalidation. I recommend it highly.

**Andrew Lotery MD FRCOphth**
**Professor of Ophthalmology**
**Southampton General Hospital, UK**
*December 2011*

# Preface

Structured examinations continue to play a large part in the assessment of ophthalmologists in training and are likely to do so for some time to come. The initial examinations that a doctor has to overcome are usually in the basic sciences and theoretical optics necessary to give a solid foundation to the clinical conditions he or she may see in the course of their training. There are precious few textbooks that allow the trainee to assess their own knowledge of basic sciences in ophthalmology. This book will, hopefully, fill the gap.

We have concentrated mainly on the first part of the FRCOphth examination held by the Royal College of Ophthalmologists and the Basic Science and Optics paper of the International Council of Ophthalmology (ICO). The book follows the multiple-choice structure of these two examinations and is aimed mainly at ophthalmologists wishing to take these examinations. However, this book is not exclusive, and trainees embarking on other ophthalmology examinations, such as the FRCS (Ophthalmology) examinations in Glasgow and Edinburgh, as well as the DRCOphth and the Duke Elder ophthalmology examination for medical students, will find it useful. In addition, more senior ophthalmologists may find it helpful in refreshing their knowledge in ophthalmic basic sciences for continuing professional development and in preparation for revalidation.

The book is divided into relevant chapters with topics that follow on logically from one another. Each chapter has multiple-choice questions in the FRCOphth format (a single best answer from a choice of four) and in the ICO format (five true or false answers). We have tried not to allow duplication of the two formats so that each question is original and all readers can benefit from all the questions. Each of the question chapters follows each other, and a separate answer section then continues. This is to allow the reader, if so desired, to treat the questions section as a real examination without having the opportunity to look at the answers. The answer sections are fully referenced to allow the reader to search further if required.

A novel feature of this book is that each question has been provided with a level-of-difficulty score. This ranges from 1 (easy) to 5 (fiendish). The scoring has been compiled using a form of modified Angoff structure. This is a well-recognised educational tool that most examination bodies employ to gauge the difficulty of individual questions. It is based on the authors of the book collectively imagining a 'minimally competent' student. This is not an average student, but one who would just scrape a pass in the examination. Each of the authors then imagines five of these students and estimates how many of them would correctly answer the particular question. The individual scores are averaged to produce an overall score for the question. The method is not foolproof, but may allow the reader to appreciate the level of difficulty of the question.

Trainee doctors in ophthalmology face a long path before they are proficient in the subject. Even then, constant updating of knowledge continues. We feel that this book will prove to be a useful tool for those preparing for the early examinations in the specialty. We wish them the very best of luck.

ST, SdS, HM, SK
*December 2011*

# About the authors

**Sameer Trikha** received academic distinctions in medicine at the University of Southampton Medical School and has since been extensively involved in medical education at undergraduate and postgraduate levels, developing teaching curricula for clinical medical students and emergency staff. As a national prize winner, he maintains a strong interest in clinical research, with numerous international presentations to his name. He has successfully completed the MRCOphth examination, and is a specialist trainee in the Wessex deanery.

**Samantha de Silva** graduated from Oxford University Medical School and undertook postgraduate training in medicine, obtaining the MRCP examination before embarking on a career in ophthalmology. She was awarded the Royal College of Ophthalmologists' Harcourt Medal for MRCOphth part 3. She is currently a specialist trainee in the Oxford deanery and a clinical research fellow at the Nuffield Laboratory of Ophthalmology, undertaking research into retinal degenerations.

**Hemal Mehta** carried out his preclinical medical training at Cambridge University, where he carried out basic sciences research on photoreceptor regeneration. He completed his clinical studies at University College London, where he was awarded the prestigious Royal College of Ophthalmologists' Duke Elder Award. He is a trainee in the London deanery and has a keen interest in medical education, recently being involved in the organisation of the inaugural Royal Society of Medicine Undergraduate Course in Ophthalmology and the Moorfields Eye Hospital A&E Course for Trainees.

The senior author, **Simon Keightley**, has been a consultant ophthalmologist at North Hampshire Hospital in Basingstoke for 21 years. For much of that time, he has been an examiner for the Royal College of Ophthalmologists. Latterly, he was senior examiner and chairman of the Examinations Committee of the

College as well as a vice-president until 2008. He has designed the restructuring of the college's examinations and other assessments in line with the Modernising Medical Careers programme and has spent many long hours ensuring that it serves well as a blueprint with the radical changes in the ophthalmic trainees' curriculum. He is now an examiner for the International Council of Ophthalmology (ICO) examinations and continues to examine for the Royal College of Ophthalmologists. Much of his time is now spent designing questions for ophthalmic examinations and General Medical Council (GMC) performance assessments.

# Acknowledgements

We are extremely grateful to the following:

Mr Simon Madge, consultant ophthalmologist at the Victoria Eye Unit, Hereford Hospitals NHS Trust, for his help and advice at the outset of this project.

Mrs Phyllis Spence, library administrator, Department of Ophthalmology at Queen Alexandra Hospital, Portsmouth Hospitals NHS Trust, for her help in sourcing references.

Our families, for their patience and support during the many hours we have spent during the writing of this book.

**ST, SdS, HM, SK**

# 1
# Anatomy

# 50 FRCOphth best-fit MCQs

1 The orbicularis oculi muscle is supplied by the:
   a. Oculomotor nerve
   b. Abducens nerve
   c. Facial nerve
   d. Glossopharyngeal nerve

2 Which of the following bones is *not* part of the medial wall of the orbit?
   a. Zygomatic
   b. Maxillary
   c. Lacrimal
   d. Ethmoid

3 The levator palpebrae superioris is supplied by which one of the following?
   a. Trochlear nerve
   b. Superior branch of the oculomotor nerve
   c. Maxillary branch of the trigeminal nerve
   d. Mandibular branch of the trigeminal nerve

4 The approximate volume of the orbit is:
   a. 60 mL
   b. 10 mL
   c. 30 mL
   d. 45 mL

5 The order of insertion of the rectus muscles from closest to furthest from the limbus is:
   a. Inferior rectus, superior rectus, medial rectus, lateral rectus
   b. Medial rectus, lateral rectus, superior rectus, inferior rectus
   c. Lateral rectus, superior rectus, medial rectus, inferior rectus
   d. Medial rectus, inferior rectus, lateral rectus, superior rectus

6 The actions of the inferior oblique are:
   a. Elevates, intorts and excyclotorts the eye
   b. Depresses, intorts and incyclotorts the eye
   c. Extorts, elevates and abducts the eye
   d. Intorts, elevates and abducts the eye

**7** The anatomical limbus is bordered anteriorly by:
 **a.** The membrane joining Bowman's line with the end of Descemet's line
 **b.** Conjunctival epithelium
 **c.** Scleral spur
 **d.** Trabecular meshwork

**8** Which of the following structures does not pass within the common tendinous ring?
 **a.** Oculomotor nerve
 **b.** Abducens nerve
 **c.** Nasociliary nerve
 **d.** Superior ophthalmic vein

**9** Which one of the following transmits the maxillary nerve?
 **a.** Foramen ovale
 **b.** Foramen of Magendie
 **c.** Foramen lacerum
 **d.** Foramen rotundum

**10** Which of the following statements is true regarding the lacrimal gland?
 **a.** The sympathetic supply arises via the deep petrosal nerve and the parasympathetic supply via the nervus intermedius
 **b.** The sympathetic supply arises via the ophthalmic nerve and the parasympathetic supply via the nervus intermedius
 **c.** The sympathetic supply arises via the ophthalmic nerve and the parasympathetic supply via the mandibular nerve
 **d.** The sympathetic supply arises via the mandibular nerve and the parasympathetic supply via the deep petrosal nerve

**11** From which of the following arteries does the pretarsal portion of the eyelid derive its arterial supply?
 **a.** The ophthalmic artery
 **b.** The maxillary artery
 **c.** The superficial temporal artery
 **d.** The meningeal artery

**12** Which of the following extraocular muscles assumes a fusiform shape?
 **a.** Inferior oblique
 **b.** Superior rectus
 **c.** Müller's muscle
 **d.** Superior oblique

13  A thickened arrangement of connective tissue bands between the inferior oblique and inferior rectus is known as:
   a. Müller's muscle
   b. The suspensory ligament of Lockwood
   c. The accessory muscle of Wolfring
   d. Periorbital fascia

14  Which of the following statements about the lacrimal caruncle is true?
   a. It contains a large amount of accessory lacrimal and sebaceous gland tissue
   b. It is highly vascular
   c. Anatomically it is situated in the lateral fornix
   d. Anatomically it is situated in the superotemporal forniceal conjunctiva

15  The following vessels are end branches of the ophthalmic artery:
   a. Dorsal nasal and supratrochlear branches
   b. Infratrochlear branch
   c. Zygomaticofacial branch
   d. Lacrimal artery branch

16  The intraorbital portion of the optic nerve is supplied by:
   a. Pial branches of the central retinal artery
   b. Circle of Zinn-Haller
   c. Peripapillary choroidal vessels
   d. Retinal arterioles

17  The superior orbital fissure does *not* transmit:
   a. The abducens nerve
   b. The trochlear nerve
   c. The oculomotor nerve
   d. The maxillary nerve

18  The canal of Schlemm:
   a. Is lined with epithelium
   b. Directly communicates with the trabecular meshwork
   c. Lies within the internal scleral sulcus
   d. Is drained by collector channels which join the major arterial circle

19 Regarding the iris:
   a. The stroma is covered by an epithelial layer anteriorly
   b. The stroma is derived from neural ectoderm
   c. The collarette is where the iris is thinnest
   d. The layer containing melanin is continuous with the inner non-pigmented ciliary epithelium

20 Regarding the innervation of the iris sphincter pupillae muscle:
   a. Parasympathetic supply is via the short ciliary nerves
   b. Sympathetic supply is via the short ciliary nerves
   c. Parasympathetic supply is via the long ciliary nerves
   d. Sympathetic supply is via the long ciliary nerves

21 With respect to the lens:
   a. It is more convex anteriorly than posteriorly
   b. It measures approximately 10 mm in diameter
   c. The capsule is thickest at the anterior and posterior poles
   d. Lens fibres are pentagonal in cross section

22 When using accommodation to focus on a near object, which of the following is true?
   a. Contraction of the meridional ciliary muscle fibres pulls the ciliary body forwards
   b. Contraction of the circular ciliary muscle fibres pulls the ciliary body outwards
   c. The tension on the zonules is increased
   d. The lens acquires a less globular shape

23 Regarding the ciliary body:
   a. It is approximately 8 mm wide
   b. The anterior surface is smooth and surrounds the periphery of the iris
   c. The posterior surface is smooth and becomes continuous with the choroid
   d. The zonules attach to the tips of the ciliary processes

24 Regarding the ciliary epithelium:
   a. The pigmented inner layer is the continuation of the retinal pigment epithelium
   b. The basement membrane of the non-pigmented cells is continuous with the inner limiting membrane of the retina
   c. The pigmented cells contain Golgi apparatus, endoplasmic reticulum and mitochondria
   d. Only the non-pigmented cells produce aqueous humour

**25** Regarding the layers of the choroid:
  **a.** The inner layer consists of connective tissue containing melanocytes
  **b.** The inner layer contains branches of the short posterior ciliary arteries
  **c.** The capillaries of the middle layer are lined with fenestrated epithelial cells
  **d.** The basement membrane of the retinal pigment epithelium is a constituent of Bruch's membrane

**26** Regarding the layers of the neurosensory retina:
  **a.** The outer plexiform layer consists of synaptic connections between bipolar, amacrine and ganglion cells
  **b.** The inner nuclear layer consists of nuclei of rod and cone cells
  **c.** The nerve fibre layer consists of axons of bipolar cells
  **d.** The inner limiting membrane consists of terminations of Müller cells and covering basement membrane

**27** Which of the following is true with respect to the optic nerve?
  **a.** The nerve fibres within the eye anterior to the optic disc are myelinated
  **b.** The optic nerve passes posteriorly through the optic canal in the greater wing of sphenoid
  **c.** The venous drainage of the orbital part of the optic nerve is into the central retinal vein
  **d.** The arterial supply of the orbital part of the optic nerve is from the central retinal artery and anterior ciliary arteries

**28** Regarding the bones of the skull:
  **a.** The frontal bone articulates with the parietal bone at the coronal suture
  **b.** The two parietal bones articulate with each other at the lamboid suture
  **c.** The parietal bone articulates with the occipital bone at the sagittal suture
  **d.** The squamous temporal bone articulates with the parietal bone at the temporal suture

**29** Regarding the meninges:
   **a.** The endosteal layer of the dura mater is continuous with the dura mater of the spinal cord
   **b.** The tentorium cerebelli is attached to the crista galli
   **c.** The subarachnoid space separates the dura and arachnoid mater
   **d.** The middle meningeal artery passes through the foramen spinosum to lie between the two layers of the dura mater

**30** Which of the following is true?
   **a.** The sella turcica is a deep depression in the body of the sphenoid bone
   **b.** The sella turcica is bounded anteriorly by the dorsum sellae
   **c.** The sphenoidal sinuses lie superiorly to the pituitary gland
   **d.** The pituitary gland lies superiorly to the optic chiasm

**31** Which of the following is true?
   **a.** The ophthalmic artery runs through the superior orbital fissure
   **b.** The mandibular nerve runs through the foramen rotundum
   **c.** The internal carotid artery runs through the foramen lacerum
   **d.** The vagus nerve runs through the foramen magnum

**32** Which of the following does *not* lie in the lateral wall of the cavernous sinus?
   **a.** Oculomotor nerve
   **b.** Trochlear nerve
   **c.** Maxillary division of the trigeminal nerve
   **d.** Optic nerve

**33** Which of the following cranial nerves is *not* affected by a cerebellopontine angle mass?
   **a.** Oculomotor nerve
   **b.** Ophthalmic division of trigeminal nerve
   **c.** Facial nerve
   **d.** Vestibulocochlear nerve

**34** Which of the following tasks would not be affected by damage to the left vagus nerve?
   **a.** Gag reflex
   **b.** Cough reflex
   **c.** Peristalsis of the small intestine
   **d.** Salivary gland secretions

**35** Which of the following parts of the cerebellum is most important to the vestibular system?
a. Vermis
b. Tonsils
c. Flocculonodular lobe
d. Middle peduncle

**36** Which of the following cell types carry efferent information from the cerebellum?
a. Climbing fibres
b. Mossy fibres
c. Purkinje cells
d. Amacrine cells

**37** Approximately what percentage of the primary visual cortex represents the macula?
a. 1%
b. 10%
c. 30%
d. 100%

**38** Which of the following sinuses does not drain into the middle meatus?
a. Frontal sinus
b. Maxillary sinus
c. Anterior group of ethmoidal sinus
d. Posterior group of ethmoidal sinus

**39** The pulmonary artery originates from which chamber of the heart?
a. Right ventricle
b. Right atrium
c. Aorta
d. Left ventricle

**40** Which of the following statements regarding the structure of blood vessels is *false*?
a. Arteries carry blood away from the heart
b. Arteries contain valves to prevent backflow
c. Arteriosclerosis describes a group of diseases characterised by thickening and loss of elasticity of the arterial walls
d. Veins are thinner walled than companion arteries

**41** Which of the following statements about lymphatic drainage from the orbit and ocular adnexa is true?
  **a.** Lymphatic vessels and nodes are present in the orbit
  **b.** Submandibular lymph nodes drain the superior aspect of periocular tissue
  **c.** Lymphatic drainage of the eyelids and conjunctiva parallels the course of arteries
  **d.** Superficial preauricular lymph nodes drain the lateral aspect of periocular tissue

**42** Which of the following statements regarding the thoracic duct is *false*?
  **a.** The thoracic duct begins at the chyle cistern in the abdomen
  **b.** The thoracic duct drains lymph for the entire body
  **c.** The thoracic duct passes anterior to the sympathetic trunk
  **d.** The thoracic duct passes posterior to the carotid sheath

**43** Which layers of the lateral geniculate nucleus receive input from the contralateral optic nerve?
  **a.** Layers 4, 5, 6
  **b.** Layers 1, 2, 3
  **c.** Layers 1, 4, 6
  **d.** Layers 2, 3, 5

**44** Which of the following provides the arterial supply to the lateral geniculate nuclei?
  **a.** Anterior choroidal and posterior cerebral arteries
  **b.** Posterior choroidal arteries
  **c.** Posterior communicating and anterior choroidal arteries
  **d.** Deep optic branch of the middle cerebral arteries

**45** Which of the following divisions of the trigeminal (fifth) cranial nerve does *not* pass through the cavernous sinus?
  **a.** Ophthalmic
  **b.** Maxillary
  **c.** Mandibular
  **d.** Maxillary and mandibular

**46** Which of the following structures passes through the annulus of Zinn?
  **a.** Frontal nerve
  **b.** Nasociliary nerve
  **c.** Trochlear nerve
  **d.** Lacrimal nerve

**47** Which of the following structures divides the two lobes of the lacrimal gland?
   a. Levator aponeurosis
   b. Orbicularis oculi
   c. Tarsal plate
   d. Superior oblique

**48** Which cranial nerve is most likely to be damaged with a closed head injury?
   a. I
   b. IV
   c. V
   d. VII

**49** Where would a lesion causing a right homonymous superotemporal quadrantanopia be localised?
   a. Left optic nerve
   b. Left optic tract
   c. Left parietal lobe
   d. Left temporal lobe

**50** What field defect would you expect to see in a patient with a lesion in their left optic tract?
   a. Right homonymous hemianiopia
   b. Left homonymous hemianopia
   c. Right homonymous inferior quadrantanopia
   d. Bitemporal quadrantanopia

# 50 ICO true/false MCQs

**51** Regarding the features of the skull, which of the following statements are true and which are false?
- i. The cranial vault consists of eight bones
- ii. Four of 14 facial bones are unpaired
- iii. The nasal cavity is important for olfaction and respiration
- iv. The frontal bone is the largest bone
- v. The occipital bone is bordered anteriorly by the parietal bone

**52** Regarding the paranasal sinuses, which of the following statements are true and which are false?
- i. The sinuses cool the brain
- ii. The frontal sinus is supplied by the supraorbital nerve
- iii. The optic chiasm lies immediately below the sphenoidal sinus
- iv. The maxillary sinus is in contact with the nasal cavity through the inferior meatus
- v. The sinuses warm and moisten air

**53** Regarding the recti muscles, which of the following statements are true and which are false?
- i. The medial rectus insertion lies 5.5 mm from the limbus
- ii. The lateral rectus insertion lies 5.5 mm from the limbus
- iii. The superior rectus muscle belly is the longest of the extraocular muscles
- iv. The superior oblique has the shortest muscle tendon
- v. The inferior oblique has the shortest muscle tendon

**54** Regarding cranial nerves, which of the following statements are true and which are false?

   i. The origin of the trochlear nerve lies at the level of the inferior colliculus

   ii. The abducens nerve origin lies in the midpons, and the fibres first pass posteriorly to emerge on the lower border of the pons above the medulla near the midline

   iii. The ophthalmic division of the trigeminal nerve represents the embryological nerve to the frontonasal swelling

   iv. The maxillary branch of the trigeminal nerve passes through the foramen ovale and traverses the pterygopalatine fossa

   v. Hutchinson's sign implies nasociliary nerve involvement in herpes zoster ophthalmicus

**55** Regarding the lacrimal apparatus, which of the following statements are true and which are false?

   i. Each canaliculus is approximately 15 mm long

   ii. The superior canaliculus has a horizontal component

   iii. The lacrimal gland is divided into a larger palpebral and smaller orbital portion

   iv. The blood supply of the lacrimal gland is from the ethmoid artery

   v. Lymphatic drainage from the lacrimal gland occurs via the preauricular lymph node

**56** Regarding the visual pathway, which of the following statements are true and which are false?

   i. The optic chiasm usually lies behind the optic groove, in front of and above the tuber cinereum.

   ii. The optic tracts divide into two sections around the rostral midbrain, a smaller lateral part and a larger medial part

   iii. The lateral geniculate nucleus (LGN) consists of eight laminae orientated in a dome-shaped mound

   iv. Geniculocalcarine tracts wind in varying degrees around the tip of the lateral ventricle

   v. Nerve fibres from the nasal hemiretina do not cross the optic chiasm

**57** Regarding the corneal endothelium, which of the following statements are true and which are false?
   i. It consists of columnar epithelial cells
   ii. Corneal endothelial cells align in a triangular arrangement
   iii. Corneal endothelial cells contain relatively few mitochondria
   iv. Density below 2500 cells/mm$^3$ leads to corneal oedema
   v. Hassall-Henle excrescences are commonly visible in Avellino corneal dystrophy

**58** Regarding the layers of the retina, which of the following statements are true and which are false?
   i. The retinal pigment epithelium sits upon Bruch's membrane
   ii. The outer plexiform layer sits upon the retinal pigment epithelium, between the inner nuclear layer and the nerve fibre layer
   iii. The inner nuclear layer lies in between the inner and outer plexiform layers
   iv. The choriocapillaris sits above the ganglion cell layer
   v. The nerve fibre layer sits upon the ganglion cell layer

**59** Regarding the vasculature of the orbit, which of the following statements are true and which are false?
   i. The ophthalmic artery branches from the lacrimal artery
   ii. The ophthalmic artery divides into dorsal nasal and infratrochlear branches
   iii. The transverse facial artery anastomoses with the lacrimal artery
   iv. The central retinal artery arises from the ophthalmic artery
   v. The retina is nourished by the central retinal artery alone

**60** Regarding the blood supply to the retina, which of the following statements are true and which are false?
   i. The retina has the highest oxygen consumption of any tissue in the human body, by weight
   ii. The blood-retinal barrier is relatively weak
   iii. The inner two-thirds of the retina are nourished by the choroidal circulation
   iv. The central retinal artery passes alongside the central retinal vein as it passes forwards in the optic nerve
   v. The central retinal artery resembles other muscular arteries and can be affected by giant cell (temporal) arteritis

**61** Regarding the optic nerve, which of the following statements are true and which are false?

  i. Foveal and macula fibres account for about 90% of all axons leaving the eye and form the distinct maculopapillary bundle

  ii. The intraocular portion of the nerve is the longest

  iii. The intraocular portion carries myelinated nerve fibres

  iv. The absence of retinal tissue around the optic nerve explains the blind spot phenomenon

  v. The intracranial portion of the nerve is damaged in glaucoma

**62** Regarding the retinal pigment epithelium, which of the following statements are true and which are false?

  i. Apical microvilli are absent

  ii. Junctional complexes are important to maintain the blood-retinal barrier

  iii. Smooth endoplasmic reticulum is absent but rough endoplasmic reticulum is present in high concentrations

  iv. Few mitochondria are present

  v. Lysosomes are present for digesting photoreceptor disks

**63** Regarding aqueous outflow, which of the following statements are true and which are false?

  i. Schlemm's canal lies on the inner aspect of the trabecular meshwork

  ii. The base of the trabecular meshwork is formed posteriorly by the scleral spur

  iii. The apex of the trabecular meshwork terminates anteriorly at Schwalbe's line

  iv. Aqueous humour passes between the intertrabecular spaces only

  v. The canal of Schlemm is not drained by aqueous veins

**64** Regarding rods and cones, which of the following statements are true and which are false?

  i. Rods contain the visual pigment rhodopsin

  ii. Cones are longer in length compared to rods

  iii. Cones synapse with bipolar and horizontal cells

  iv. Cones and rods are present at the fovea

  v. Cone lamellae are surrounded by plasma membrane

**65** Regarding the oculomotor nerve, which of the following statements are true and which are false?
   i. The Edinger-Westphal nucleus contains sympathetic nerve fibres
   ii. The oculomotor nuclei lie at the level of the superior colliculus
   iii. As the nerve traverses forward, it passes between the posterior cerebral artery and the posterior cerebellar artery
   iv. The nerve runs in the lower medial wall of the cavernous sinus
   v. The nerve enters the orbit through the inferior orbital fissure

**66** Regarding reflexes involving the facial nerve, which of the following statements are true and which are false?
   i. The afferent pathway for the corneal reflex is the long ciliary nerves
   ii. The effector muscle of the loud noise reflex is the medial pterygoid muscle
   iii. The efferent pathway of the corneal touch reflex is the temporal and zygomatic branches of the facial nerve
   iv. The receptors for the blinking to bright light reflex are the retinal cones
   v. The afferent pathway for the loud noise reflex is the vestibulocochlear nerve

**67** Regarding the muscles of the eye, which of the following statements are true and which are false?
   i. The levator palpebrae superioris is innervated by the trochlear nerve
   ii. The medial rectus is innervated by the abducens nerve
   iii. The lateral rectus is innervated by the abducens nerve
   iv. The inferior oblique is innervated by the trochlear nerve
   v. The superior oblique is innervated by the trochlear nerve

**68** Regarding the walls of the orbit, which of the following statements are true and which are false?
   i. The medial wall is formed by the lacrimal bone, ethmoid, lesser wing of sphenoid and frontal process of the maxilla
   ii. The orbital floor is formed by the orbital plate of the maxilla, orbital surface of the zygoma and the palatine bone
   iii. The lateral wall is formed by the lesser wing of sphenoid bone and the zygomatic bone
   iv. The roof of the orbit is formed by the frontal bone and the greater wing of sphenoid
   v. The roof of the orbit is formed by the frontal bone and the lesser wing of the sphenoid

**69** Regarding the middle cranial fossa, which of the following statements are true and which are false?
   i. The foramen ovale transmits the middle meningeal artery
   ii. The foramen lacerum transmits the middle meningeal artery
   iii. The foramen rotundum transmits the maxillary nerve
   iv. The foramen lacerum transmits sympathetic nerves
   v. The foramen spinosum transmits the middle meningeal artery

**70** With reference to the uveal tract, which of the following statements are true and which are false?
   i. It consists of the iris and ciliary body only
   ii. The iris is 8 mm in diameter
   iii. The iris dilator pupillae is innervated by sympathetic fibres
   iv. The iris is supplied by the posterior ciliary arteries
   v. The iris is innervated by branches of the inferior orbital nerve

**71** With reference to the cornea, which of the following statements are true and which are false?
   i. The corneal stroma consists of irregularly orientated collagen lamellae
   ii. The corneal stroma contains mainly collagen type 1
   iii. Bowman's layer consists of regularly arranged collagen fibres
   iv. The corneal epithelium is rich in immunocompetent cells
   v. Descemet's membrane is 8–12 µm in thickness

**72** Regarding the lens, which of the following statements are true and which are false?
   i. In the adult the lens has an axial length of approximately 2 mm
   ii. The lens capsule consists of glycoproteins
   iii. Lens epithelium consists of simple stratified squamous epithelium
   iv. Numerous gap junctions exist between cells in the lens
   v. Lens fibres are rich in cytoskeletal elements

**73** Regarding the vitreous, which of the following statements are true and which are false?
   i. The posterior depression is known as the hyaloid fossa
   ii. The central vitreous contains tightly packed collagen
   iii. The vitreous base is a tight 3- to 4-mm band
   iv. The ligamentum hyaloide capsulare is attached to the optic disc
   v. The vitreous is adherent to the optic disc

**74** With reference to the ciliary body, which of the following statements are true and which are false?

    i. It separates the scleral spur from the ora serrata

    ii. The base faces the anterior chamber

    iii. The pars plana is a 6-mm zone

    iv. Longitudinal muscle fibres are attached to the scleral spur

    v. The ora serrata contains pigmented ciliary epithelium

**75** With reference to the ciliary body, which of the following statements are true and which are false?

    i. The blood supply is from the short posterior ciliary arteries

    ii. The blood supply is from the long posterior ciliary arteries

    iii. The parasympathetic innervation is via the Edinger-Westphal nucleus

    iv. Preganglionic sympathetic nerve fibres are situated at T1 in the spinal cord

    v. Preganglionic sympathetic nerve fibres are situated at C5 in the spinal cord

**76** Regarding the internal carotid artery, which of the following statements are true and which are false?

    i. The ophthalmic artery arises from the internal carotid artery

    ii. The vidian artery (artery of the pterygoid canal) arises from the internal carotid artery

    iii. The posterior cerebellar artery arises from the internal carotid artery

    iv. The superior hypophyseal artery arises from the ophthalmic artery

    v. The middle cerebral artery arises from the ophthalmic artery

**77** Regarding the superior rectus, which of the following statements are true and which are false?

    i. The superior rectus originates from a common tendinous ring

    ii. The superior rectus is innervated by the 3rd cranial nerve

    iii. The length of the muscle belly is approximately 41 mm

    iv. The length of the muscle belly is approximately 31 mm

    v. The insertion of the superior rectus is 7.8 mm from the cornea

**78** Regarding the facial nerve, which of the following statements are true and which are false?

  **i.** It exits the skull from the stylomastoid foramen
  **ii.** It exits the skull from the foramen rotundum
  **iii.** It arises from the 1st pharyngeal arch
  **iv.** It arises from the 2nd pharyngeal arch
  **v.** It supplies the stapedius muscle

**79** Regarding the muscles of the face, which of the following statements are true and which are false?

  **i.** The galea aponeurotica attaches the frontal bellies to the occipital bellies of the occipitofrontalis muscle
  **ii.** The galea intermedia attaches the frontal bellies to the occipital bellies of the occipitofrontalis muscle
  **iii.** Depressor supercilii fibres of the orbicularis oculi are inserted in the skin of the eyebrow
  **iv.** Elevator supercilii fibres of the orbicularis oculi are inserted in the skin of the eyebrow
  **v.** The levator palpebrae superioris originates from the lesser wing of sphenoid

**80** Regarding the lacrimal gland, which of the following statements are true and which are false?

  **i.** It is supplied by the lacrimal artery
  **ii.** It is supplied by the infraorbital artery
  **iii.** It is drained by the ophthalmic veins
  **iv.** It is drained by the vortex veins
  **v.** It is supplied by the sympathetic nervous system

**81** Regarding the blood supply to the visual pathway, which of the following statements are true and which are false?

  **i.** The optic chiasm is supplied by the superior hypophyseal artery
  **ii.** The lateral geniculate nucleus is supplied by the posterior cerebellar artery
  **iii.** The lateral geniculate nucleus is supplied by the anterior choroidal artery
  **iv.** The optic radiation is supplied by the anterior choroidal artery
  **v.** The optic radiation is supplied by the superior hypophyseal artery

**82** Regarding the eyelids, which of the following statements are true and which are false?

i. The lymphatic drainage of the eyelids involves the superficial parotid nodes

ii. The lymphatic drainage of the eyelids involves the submental lymph nodes

iii. The pretarsal portion of the eyelid is supplied by facial arteries

iv. The post-tarsal portion of the eyelid is supplied by facial arteries

v. Post-tarsal venous drainage is via the ophthalmic veins

**83** Regarding the blood supply of the orbit, which of the following statements are true and which are false?

i. The posterior ciliary arteries divide into four short and four long posterior ciliary arteries

ii. The ophthalmic artery arises from the internal carotid artery

iii. The ophthalmic artery divides into the dorsal nasal and trochlear arteries

iv. The lacrimal artery is derived from the facial artery

v. The veins in the orbits have numerous valves

**84** Regarding the primary visual cortex, which of the following statements are true and which are false?

i. It is situated either side of the calcarine sulcus

ii. Input is primarily from the contralateral lateral geniculate nucleus

iii. The macula projects anteriorly and the peripheral retina posteriorly

iv. Only cells after the first synapse in the primary visual cortex receive binocular input

v. Layer V projects to the superior colliculus

**85** Regarding saccadic eye movements, which of the following statements are true and which are false?

i. Saccadic eye movements are the fastest of eye movements

ii. The maximum saccadic velocity is 20 degrees per second

iii. Horizontal saccades are controlled by the frontal eye fields

iv. The parapontine reticular formation is the start of the final common pathway of horizontal eye movements

v. Vertical saccades are generated in the rostral interstitial nucleus of the medial longitudinal fasciculus

86  Regarding the 4th (trochlear) cranial nerve, which of the following statements are true and which are false?
    i. The trochlear is the only cranial nerve to leave the brainstem dorsally
    ii. The medial longitudinal fasciculus links the 4th nerve nucleus to the nuclei of the 3rd, 6th and 8th cranial nerves
    iii. The trochlear nerve passes forwards in the medial wall of the cavernous sinus
    iv. The trochlear nerve passes inside the annulus of Zinn
    v. The trochlear nerve supplies the superior oblique muscle

87  Regarding the 6th (abducens) cranial nerve, which of the following statements are true and which are false?
    i. The abducens nerve has motor and sensory components
    ii. The nucleus of the abducens nerve is situated in the floor of the fourth ventricle
    iii. Within the cavernous sinus, the abducens nerve runs inferolateral to the internal carotid artery
    iv. The abducens nerve enters the orbit through the superior orbital fissure
    v. The abducens nerve innervates the medial rectus muscle

88  Regarding the lymphatic drainage of the head and neck, which of the following statements are true and which are false?
    i. All lymphatic drainage from the head and neck goes to the inferior deep cervical lymph nodes
    ii. Lymphatic vessels in the eyelids follow the course of the corresponding veins
    iii. Lymphatic vessels in the eyelids drain to the preauricular and submandibular lymph nodes
    iv. Lymph from the orbit drains to the superficial cervical lymph nodes
    v. Lymphatic follicles lie at the centre of lymph nodes

89  Regarding the lateral geniculate nucleus (LGN), which of the following statements are true and which are false?
    i. The internal capsule is medial to the LGN
    ii. The LGN has four layers of grey matter
    iii. Layers 1 and 2 of the LGN contribute to the magnocellular pathway
    iv. Each lamina of the LGN receives input from one eye only
    v. The majority of the fibres from the LGN pass on to the optic radiation

**90** Regarding the 7th (facial) cranial nerve, which of the following statements are true and which are false?

   **i.** It supplies muscles of facial expression

   **ii.** It supplies muscles of mastication

   **iii.** It supplies sensation to the posterior third of the tongue

   **iv.** It supplies sensation to the external auditory canal

   **v.** It supplies parasympathetic innervation to the lacrimal gland

**91** Regarding the visual pathway, which of the following statements are true and which are false?

   **i.** Lesions of the left nasal retina cause homonymous field defects

   **ii.** Lesions of the optic nerve cause homonymous field defects

   **iii.** Lesions of the optic chiasm cause homonymous field defects

   **iv.** Lesions of the optic tract cause homonymous field defects

   **v.** Lesions of Meyer's loop in the temporal lobe cause homonymous field defects

**92** Regarding the autonomic nervous system, which of the following statements are true and which are false?

   **i.** Sympathetic fibres leave the spinal cord through the ventral roots

   **ii.** Parasympathetic fibres in the short ciliary nerve are preganglionic

   **iii.** Postganglionic sympathetic supply passes to the eye only via the long ciliary nerves

   **iv.** The sympathetic supply to the eye originates from T1–T2

   **v.** Sympathetic fibres originate in the anterior horn of the spinal cord

**93** Regarding the trigeminal nerve, which of the following statements are true and which are false?

   **i.** Both the trigeminal and facial nuclei are situated in the pons

   **ii.** The spinal nerve is responsible for tactile sensation

   **iii.** The nasociliary branch passes through the annulus of Zinn

   **iv.** The lacrimal branch lies above the superior rectus muscle

   **v.** The course of the trigeminal nerve runs over the facial and auditory nerves in the posterior fossa

**94** Regarding parasympathetic nuclei, which of the following statements are true and which are false?

   **i.** The superior salivatory nucleus supplies fibres to the submandibular and sublingual glands

   **ii.** The superior salivatory nucleus supplies fibres to the parotid gland

   **iii.** The inferior salivatory nucleus supplies fibres to the lacrimal gland

   **iv.** The dorsal motor vagal nucleus supplies fibres to the gastrointestinal tract

   **v.** The Edinger-Westphal nucleus supplies fibres to the sphincter pupillae

**95** Regarding the position of the optic chiasm, which of the following statements are true and which are false?

   **i.** The optic chiasm lies lateral to the cavernous sinus

   **ii.** The optic chiasm lies inferior to the internal carotid

   **iii.** The optic chiasm lies superior to the third ventricle

   **iv.** The optic chiasm lies anterior to the cerebral arteries

   **v.** The optic chiasm lies inferior to the anterior communicating artery

**96** Regarding the carotid arteries, which of the following statements are true and which are false?

   **i.** Both carotid arteries arise from the aortic arch

   **ii.** The common carotid arteries bifurcate at the level of the third cervical vertebrae

   **iii.** The internal carotid artery has no branches in the neck

   **iv.** The internal carotid artery enters the parotid gland

   **v.** The superficial temporal artery is a terminal branch of the external carotid artery

**97** Regarding ocular dominance columns, which of the following statements are true and which are false?

   **i.** The visual cortex shows columnar organisation

   **ii.** Ocular dominance columns from each eye lie next to each other

   **iii.** Ocular dominance columns are arranged in a whorl-like pattern

   **iv.** Ocular dominance columns are present for the entire visual field

   **v.** With normal visual development, the area of ocular dominance columns representing each eye is equal

**98** Regarding projections from the visual cortex, which of the following statements are true and which are false?
   i. There are direct projections from the visual cortex to the frontal eye field
   ii. There are direct projections from the visual cortex to the lateral geniculate nucleus
   iii. There are direct projections from the visual cortex to the retina
   iv. There are direct projections from the visual cortex to Wernicke's area
   v. There are direct projections from the visual cortex to areas 18 and 19

**99** Regarding accommodation to a near object, which of the following statements are true and which are false?
   i. Contraction of the medial recti causes convergence of the ocular axes
   ii. The ciliary muscles relax
   iii. The pupils dilate
   iv. The lens thickens
   v. Postganglionic sympathetic fibres supply the ciliary muscles and sphincter pupillae

**100** Regarding the venous drainage of the orbit, which of the following statements are true and which are false?
   i. The venous system runs parallel to the arterial system
   ii. Valves prevent backflow
   iii. The anterior venous system has connections with the angular vein
   iv. The pterygoid plexus receives blood from the inferior ophthalmic vein
   v. The cavernous sinus receives blood from the superior ophthalmic vein, a branch of the inferior ophthalmic vein and central retinal vein

# 2
# Physiology

# 50 FRCOphth best-fit MCQs

1 The volume of plasma water of a 70-kg man is approximately:
   a. 3 L
   b. 9 L
   c. 11 L
   d. 28 L

2 The concentration of potassium in intracellular fluid is approximately:
   a. 4 mmol/L
   b. 12 mmol/L
   c. 120 mmol/L
   d. 140 mmol/L

3 The ion that contributes most to the resting membrane potential of a nerve fibre is:
   a. Sodium
   b. Potassium
   c. Chloride
   d. Calcium

4 Which of the following ions is most important for the release of vesicles containing neurotransmitter at the presynaptic nerve terminal?
   a. Sodium
   b. Potassium
   c. Chloride
   d. Calcium

5 Which of the following white blood cells is involved in combating parasitic infection?
   a. Neutrophils
   b. Eosinophils
   c. Basophils
   d. Monocytes

6  Presence of which of the following in vivo is *not* prothrombotic?
   a. Factor V Leiden
   b. Lupus anticoagulant
   c. Protein C
   d. Increased levels of homocysteine

7  In autoregulation of blood flow to organs, which of the following leads to vasoconstriction (excluding in the pulmonary vasculature)?
   a. Reduction in oxygen concentration
   b. Reduction in pH
   c. Increase in carbon dioxide concentration
   d. Increased blood pressure

8  Which of the following leads to a decrease in blood pressure?
   a. Increased end systolic volume
   b. Increased heart rate
   c. Increased cardiac output
   d. Increased total peripheral resistance

9  Vital capacity is:
   a. The sum of total lung capacity and residual volume
   b. The difference between total lung capacity and residual volume
   c. The sum of tidal volume and inspiratory reserve volume
   d. The difference between tidal volume and inspiratory reserve volume

10  Which of the following causes a shift in the oxygen-haemoglobin dissociation curve to the left?
   a. Hyperthermia
   b. Acidosis
   c. Carboxyhaemoglobin
   d. Increased $pCO_2$

11  Which of the following is a hormone synthesised by the pituitary gland?
   a. Growth hormone-releasing hormone
   b. Adrenocorticotrophic hormone
   c. Oxytocin
   d. Antidiuretic hormone

12  Which of the following is true regarding insulin?
   a. It promotes glycogen breakdown in the liver
   b. It promotes glucose entry into cells
   c. It is produced by alpha cells in the islets of Langerhans
   d. It promotes lipolysis

**13** Which of the following is *not* true regarding vitamin deficiencies?
   **a.** Vitamin A deficiency is associated with dry eye
   **b.** Vitamin $B_1$ deficiency is associated with ophthalmoplegia
   **c.** Vitamin $B_{12}$ deficiency is associated with optic atrophy
   **d.** Vitamin K deficiency is associated with increased risk of thrombosis

**14** Regarding aldosterone:
   **a.** It is produced by the zona glomerulosa of the adrenal gland
   **b.** It causes sodium excretion
   **c.** Excess secretion may cause hyperkalaemia
   **d.** It acts on the proximal tubule of the nephron

**15** Which of the following is the neurotransmitter present in autonomic ganglia?
   **a.** GABA
   **b.** Glycine
   **c.** Acetylcholine
   **d.** Noradrenaline

**16** Regarding pepsin, which of the following statements is true?
   **a.** It is secreted in the oesophagus
   **b.** It is secreted in its inactive proenzyme form, pepsinogen
   **c.** It is secreted in its active form, pepsinogen
   **d.** It is secreted in response to sympathetic stimulation

**17** Which of the following is the normal serum platelet level?
   **a.** $1–4 \times 10^9/L$
   **b.** $15–40 \times 10^9/L$
   **c.** $150–400 \times 10^9/L$
   **d.** $1500–4000 \times 10^8/L$

**18** Regarding melatonin, which of the following is true?
   **a.** It is produced by the pineal gland
   **b.** It is produced by the liver
   **c.** It is produced by the small intestine
   **d.** It is produced by the kidney

**19** Which of the following is the single most important factor in maintaining corneal transparency?
   **a.** Endothelial pump
   **b.** Constant refractive index of all layers
   **c.** Relative acellularity and matrix organisation
   **d.** Tear film

**20** Glucose metabolism in the lens principally occurs by:
   **a.** Anaerobic glycolysis
   **b.** Aerobic metabolism
   **c.** Hexose monophosphate shunt
   **d.** Sorbitol pathway

**21** When produced, aqueous humour passes out through the membranes of:
   **a.** Trabecular meshwork
   **b.** Corneal endothelial cells
   **c.** Non-pigmented cells of the ciliary body
   **d.** Pigmented cells of the ciliary body

**22** The principle of intraocular pressure measurement is defined by:
   **a.** Schwalbe's equation
   **b.** Poiseuille's law
   **c.** Imbert-Fick principle
   **d.** Holladay's equation

**23** The corneal stroma is mainly composed of which of the following?
   **a.** Keratan sulphate
   **b.** Chondroitin phosphate
   **c.** It is acellular
   **d.** Chondroitin sulphate

**24** Which of the following is *not* a physiological property of the vitreous?
   **a.** Transmits 85% of light of wavelength 300–1400 nm
   **b.** Prevents the globe from collapsing
   **c.** Refractive index of 1.66
   **d.** Allows accumulation of waste products such as lactic acid which can
       be toxic to the retina

**25** Which of the following is *not* a function of the retinal pigment epithelium?
   **a.** Secretion of mucopolysaccharide
   **b.** It plays a role in the embryological development of photoreceptors
   **c.** Absorption of stray light
   **d.** Adherence to other RPE cells via zona adherens to form the blood-
       retinal barrier

26  In phototransduction, activation of rhodopsin occurs via:
  a. Isomerisation of retinol
  b. Glycosylation of transducin
  c. Opening of GLUT-1 receptors
  d. Unfolding of opsin

27  Which of the following neuromodulators does *not* exert an effect in the retina?
  a. Thyrotropin-releasing hormone
  b. Taurine
  c. Insulin
  d. Glucagon

28  Within the retina, dopamine is present in:
  a. Amacrine cells
  b. Retinal pigment epithelium
  c. Müller cells
  d. Ganglion cells

29  Which of the following receptors suppresses aqueous outflow?
  a. α-2 agonists
  b. β-adrenergic agonists
  c. Muscarinic antagonists
  d. Cholinergic antagonists

30  The Bezold-Brücke phenomenon describes which of the following?
  a. All hues appear yellow-white as the luminosity increases
  b. All hues appear yellow-white as the luminosity decreases
  c. All hues appear achromatic as the intensity increases
  d. All hues appear achromatic as the intensity decreases

31  A number of corresponding points on the retina that project to a definite single point in space is known as:
  a. The Auberg phenomenon
  b. A horopter
  c. Panum's area
  d. The Pulfrich phenomenon

32  Saccadic-type eye movements are initiated by:
  a. The oculomotor cerebellar centre
  b. Abducent nerve nucleus
  c. Trochlear nerve nucleus
  d. The temporal cortex

**33** Motion blindness occurs as a result of:
 a. Lesions in the frontal lobe
 b. Lesions in the temporal gyrus
 c. Lesions in the superior temporal sulcus
 d. Lesions in the inferior temporal sulcus

**34** In light conditions, the resting potential of the eye is approximately:
 a. 40 mV
 b. 20 mV
 c. 10 mV
 d. 60 mV

**35** Which of the following statements about colour discrimination is true?
 a. It is poorest at long wavelengths
 b. It is affected by the distribution of rods
 c. It is maximal at the fovea
 d. It is best for short wavelengths

**36** The gene for blue cone pigment (short wavelength) is found on which chromosome?
 a. X chromosome
 b. Y chromosome
 c. Chromosome 7
 d. Chromosome 18

**37** Which of the following is *not* a monocular depth clue?
 a. Superimposed objects
 b. Linear perspective
 c. Angle of image disparity
 d. Light and shadow

**38** What percentage of ganglion cell axons pass within the parvocellular pathway?
 a. 20%
 b. 40%
 c. 60%
 d. 80%

**39** Which of the following statements about saccadic eye movements is accurate?
   a. They are under supranuclear contralateral control
   b. They are reflex movements only
   c. Their latency is less than 50 ms
   d. Saccades are the slowest of all eye movements

**40** Which of the following statements about smooth pursuit movements is not accurate?
   a. Smooth pursuit is stimulated by retinal slip
   b. They are possible if object is moving at a velocity of 30 degrees per second
   c. They are under supranuclear ipsilateral cortical control
   d. Their latency is approximately 150 ms

**41** What is the minimum threshold of Vernier hyperacuity?
   a. 1 second of arc
   b. 10 seconds of arc
   c. 30 seconds of arc
   d. 1 minute of arc

**42** Where is the physiological blind spot relative to the centre of the visual field?
   a. Superior
   b. Inferior
   c. Nasal
   d. Temporal

**43** Which of the following statements about Adie's tonic pupil is most accurate?
   a. It is more common in the elderly
   b. There is a male predilection
   c. There is slow redilation after near effort
   d. It is always unilateral

**44** During caloric testing, cold water is irrigated in the right ear. Which direction is the fast phase of nystagmus?
   a. Up
   b. Down
   c. Left
   d. Right

**45** Which of the following is *not* involved with vertical saccades?
  **a.** Frontal eye fields
  **b.** Paramedian pontine reticular formation
  **c.** Trochlear nucleus
  **d.** Oculomotor nucleus

**46** Uhthoff's phenomenon describes:
  **a.** An inability to distinguish faces
  **b.** A decrease in vision with increase in temperature
  **c.** Skew eye movements
  **d.** A decrease in vision on neck flexion

**47** Which of the following statements regarding the pattern electroretinogram (ERG) is not accurate?
  **a.** The pattern ERG represents retinal ganglion cell activity
  **b.** The $P_{50}$ component is always affected in macula disease
  **c.** The $N_{95}$ component corresponds to ganglion cell activity
  **d.** The pattern ERG is always affected in optic nerve disease

**48** Regarding a relative afferent pupillary defect, which of the following statements is accurate?
  **a.** It cannot be tested if one pupil is pharmacologically dilated
  **b.** It cannot be tested if both pupils are pharmacologically dilated
  **c.** It is likely to occur with a cataract
  **d.** It is always associated with anisocoria

**49** Which of the following methods can be used to isolate a cone response from the electroretinogram?
  **a.** Dim background lighting conditions
  **b.** 50-Hz flicker
  **c.** 10-Hz flicker
  **d.** Single-flash ERG

**50** Regarding visual evoked potentials (VEPs), which of the following statements is not accurate?
  **a.** VEPs are a measure of the response of the occipital cortex to visual stimulation
  **b.** VEPs can be used to assess crossover of visual pathway fibres at the optic chiasm
  **c.** An amblyopic eye will usually have an abnormal pattern and flash VEP
  **d.** VEPs can be used to approximate visual acuity

# 50 ICO true/false MCQs

**51** Regarding vitamin A:
  i. It is a fat-soluble vitamin
  ii. The provitamin is found in green vegetables
  iii. The provitamin is converted into retinol in the small intestine
  iv. It may be stored in the liver
  v. Xerosis is a feature of vitamin A deficiency

**52** Which of the following are associated with a reduced progression of age-related macular degeneration?
  i. Magnesium
  ii. Beta-carotene
  iii. Vitamin A
  iv. Vitamin C
  v. Vitamin E

**53** Which of the following may be seen in hyperthyroidism?
  i. Elevated thyroid-stimulating hormone (TSH), elevated free $T_4$
  ii. Suppressed TSH, elevated free $T_4$
  iii. Elevated thyroid-stimulating hormone, reduced free $T_4$
  iv. Suppressed thyroid-stimulating hormone, reduced free $T_4$
  v. Positive antithyroid peroxidase antibody

**54** Regarding oncotic pressure, which of the following statements are true and which are false?
  i. Oncotic pressure is synonymous with osmotic pressure
  ii. Albumin contributes to oncotic pressure
  iii. 80% of oncotic pressure is due to plasma globulins
  iv. Sodium ions contribute to oncotic pressure
  v. The oncotic pressure of plasma is around 29 mmHg

**55** Regarding the structure of skeletal muscle:
  i. The sarcolemma is the cell membrane of the muscle fibre
  ii. Myofibrils consist of thin myosin filaments and thick actin filaments
  iii. I bands consist of myosin filaments only
  iv. Actin filaments are attached to the Z disc
  v. The distance between two Z discs defines the sarcomere

**56** Regarding muscle contraction, which of the following statements are true and which are false?

    i. Acetylcholine (ACh) is released from the motor nerve terminal

    ii. ACh binds to muscarinic ACh receptors on the motor end plate

    iii. Potassium influx into the muscle fibre initiates an action potential

    iv. Depolarisation as a result of the action potential causes calcium release from the mitochondria

    v. Calcium binds to troponin C on the actin filaments and initiates sliding of the actin and myosin filaments

**57** Which of the following may cause haemolytic anaemia?

    i. Folate deficiency

    ii. Hereditary spherocytosis

    iii. Malaria

    iv. Glucose-6-phosphate deficiency

    v. Sickle-cell disease

**58** The following factors increase the rate of blood flow through a vessel, true or false?

    i. Smaller blood vessel diameter

    ii. Smaller difference in pressure between the ends of the vessel

    iii. Longer vessel length

    iv. Higher blood viscosity

    v. Thickness of vessel wall

**59** Regarding synaptic transmission, which of the following statements are true and which are false?

    i. The presynaptic membrane contains voltage-gated sodium channels

    ii. Adrenaline is a neurotransmitter released by the presynaptic terminal

    iii. Postsynaptic receptors are always ion channels

    iv. Sodium influx into the postsynaptic cell is excitatory

    v. Potassium influx into the postsynaptic cell is excitatory

**60** Regarding pain, which of the following statements are true and which are false?

    i. Pain receptors are free nerve endings

    ii. Mechanical and chemical stimuli only are able to activate pain receptors

    iii. Bradykinin excites pain receptors

    iv. Prostaglandins excite pain receptors

    v. Pain receptors show adaptation with loss of sensitivity with repeated stimulation

**61** Regarding tear production:
   i. Basal secretion of tears occurs via a sodium/potassium ATPase pump
   ii. The rate of basal tear secretion is 20 μl/min
   iii. Stimulated tear secretion occurs via acetylcholine release stimulating muscarinic acetylcholine receptors
   iv. The accessory lacrimal glands constantly produce tears
   v. Conjunctival sac volume is 25–30 μl

**62** Regarding the vitreous, which of the following statements are true and which are false?
   i. It contains hyaluronic acid
   ii. It contains ascorbic acid
   iii. It contains type II collagen
   iv. The central region of the vitreous contains more collagen than the cortex
   v. The vitreous in children is more liquid than that in adults

**63** Regarding the choroid, which of the following statements are true and which are false?
   i. It consists of the vessel layer, capillary layer and Bowman's membrane
   ii. It is thickest anteriorly
   iii. Its main blood supply is from the posterior ciliary arteries
   iv. It supplies the inner retina with nutrients
   v. Pigment cells in the choroid absorb excess light that has passed through the retina

**64** Regarding the blood-ocular barrier, which of the following statements are true and which are false?
   i. It consists of the blood-aqueous and blood-vitreous barriers
   ii. Ocular inflammation may breach the blood-ocular barrier
   iii. The blood-aqueous barrier is formed by tight junctions between pigmented ciliary epithelial cells
   iv. The outer retina is protected by tight junctions between retinal pigment epithelial cells
   v. The inner retina is protected by tight junctions between the endothelial cells of capillaries

**65** Regarding sympathetic stimulation of the heart, which of the following statements are true and which are false?
  **i.** Noradrenaline is the major transmitter involved
  **ii.** There is increased calcium permeability of the muscle fibre membrane
  **iii.** The rate of sinus node discharge is reduced
  **iv.** The rate of conduction within the heart is reduced
  **v.** Force of contraction is reduced

**66** Regarding photoreceptor cells, which of the following statements are true and which are false?
  **i.** They depolarise due to the closure of sodium channels
  **ii.** They hyperpolarise due to the closure of sodium channels
  **iii.** They hyperpolarise due to the closure of NMDA receptors
  **iv.** They depolarise via the closure of NMDA receptors
  **v.** They are induced by kappa receptors

**67** Regarding saccadic eye movements, which of the following statements are true and which are false?
  **i.** Rapid eye movements (REM) are an example of saccadic eye movements
  **ii.** Fast-phase nystagmus is an example of saccadic eye movements
  **iii.** Voluntary refixation is an example of saccadic eye movements
  **iv.** Optokinetic nystagmus is an example of saccadic eye movements
  **v.** Vestibular nystagmus is not an example of saccadic eye movements

**68** Regarding photoreceptors, which of the following statements are true and which are false?
  **i.** Photoreceptors have two sections
  **ii.** The cell bodies of photoreceptors lie in the inner nuclear layer
  **iii.** The inner segment connects the outer segment to the cell body within the retina
  **iv.** Eight pairs of microtubules lie within the ciliary stalk
  **v.** The ellipsoid region contains a high concentration of mitochondria

**69** Regarding human tears, which of the following statements are true and which are false?
  **i.** The pH of tears is 6.0
  **ii.** The pH of tears is 7.4
  **iii.** The refractive index of tears is 1.357
  **iv.** Tears do not contain ammonia
  **v.** Tears do not contain albumin

**70** Regarding the lens, which of the following statements are true and which are false?

   i. The lens is normally in a dehydrated state *in vivo*

   ii. Glucose is metabolised in the lens to generate ATP

   iii. Amino acids diffuse passively into the lens

   iv. Glutathione is the most actively transported amino acid into the lens

   v. Lipids represent 10%–12% of the lens

**71** Regarding the retina, which of the following statements are true and which are false?

   i. Amacrine I cells release the neurotransmitter glycine

   ii. Amacrine cells release the neurotransmitter dopamine

   iii. Amacrine II cells form gap junctions

   iv. Ganglion cells determine the spatial resolution of the visual system

   v. NMDA is the most concentrated transmitter in the retina

**72** Regarding luminosity, which of the following statements are true and which are false?

   i. In scotopic conditions, light has a peak luminosity in the 500-nm region

   ii. Under photopic conditions, light appears brightest in the 650-nm region

   iii. The Purkinje shift occurs when rod function is initiated in dark adapted conditions

   iv. Cone-specific spectral curves can be detected by desensitising rods to blue wavelength light

   v. Flicker photometry is used to measure brightness curves for cones

**73** Regarding accommodation, which of the following statements are true and which are false?

   i. The pupil constricts

   ii. The accommodation is dependent upon convergence

   iii. The anterior chamber deepens

   iv. The anterior surface of the lens becomes concave

   v. The diameter of the lens decreases

**74** Regarding aqueous humor, which of the following statements are true and which are false?

   i. The concentration of urea is higher in the aqueous than in the blood
   ii. Ascorbic acid is not present
   iii. Chloride concentrations are lower in aqueous compared with plasma
   iv. IgG levels are higher in aqueous compared with plasma
   v. Fibronectin levels are lower in aqueous compared with plasma

**75** Regarding the lens, which of the following statements are true and which are false?

   i. Lens zonules attach the ciliary processes to the lens
   ii. The posterior capsule separates the lens cortex from the aqueous humor
   iii. The lens epithelium has the highest metabolic rate
   iv. Glycosidase enzymes enable turnover of the lens capsule
   v. The lens epithelium consists of a cuboidal layer of cells

**76** Regarding light detection, which of the following statements are true and which are false?

   i. Luminance can be measured in trolands
   ii. Luminance can be measured in candelas
   iii. Light of 50–150 quanta can be perceived as a discrete flash of light
   iv. Light of 5–20 quanta can be perceived as a discrete flash of light
   v. Regeneration of rhodopsin takes approximately 60 minutes

**77** Regarding the light reflex, which of the following statements are true and which are false?

   i. The afferent response commences in the optic nerve
   ii. The afferent response terminates in the pretectal nucleus
   iii. Fibres pass through the otic ganglion
   iv. Fibres pass through the Edinger-Westphal ganglion
   v. Fibres synapse in the ciliary ganglion

**78** Regarding phototransduction, which of the following statements are true and which are false?

   i. Activation of rhodopsin occurs via the isomerisation of retinol
   ii. In the resting state, the photoreceptor is relatively depolarised
   iii. All-trans-retinol attaches to rhodopsin
   iv. 11-cis-retinol binds to cellular retinaldehyde-binding protein (CRALBP)
   v. Rhodopsin is synthesised in the outer segments of the photoreceptor

**79** Regarding the electroretinogram, which of the following statements are true and which are false?
   i. The early receptor potential is detectable in eyes where the inner retina has been destroyed
   ii. The negative a-wave is generated by depolarisation of bipolar cells
   iii. The a2 component of the a-wave is generated by the cone photoreceptor
   iv. The b-wave is generated by cone photoreceptors
   v. The c-wave is generated by the retinal pigment epithelium

**80** Regarding visual evoked potentials, which of the following statements are true and which are false?
   i. The VEP records electrical activity in the temporal lobe
   ii. The VEP records electrical activity in the occipital cortex
   iii. A pattern-flash VEP correlates well with visual acuity
   iv. The flash VEP arises in area V1 of the cortex
   v. The pattern VEP arises in the V2 area of the cortex

**81** Regarding the lacrimal gland, which of the following statements are true and which are false?
   i. The lacrimal gland secretes lipid-rich material
   ii. The lacrimal gland secretes proteinaceous material
   iii. Its secretions contain high concentrations of albumin
   iv. Its secretions contain high concentrations of lysozymes
   v. Its secretions contain high concentrations of IgM82

**82** Regarding the striate cortex:
   i. The striate cortex area V5 responds to motion
   ii. The striate cortex area V1 responds to motion
   iii. The striate cortex area V4 responds to colour
   iv. Shapes of images can be detected in area V3
   v. Shapes of images can be detected in area V5

**83** Regarding the Snellen chart, which of the following statements are true and which are false?
   i. The scale is directly proportional to the minimal angle of resolution
   ii. Each character has six elements
   iii. Each element represents 1 minute of arc
   iv. Each character represents 6 minutes of arc
   v. Each line has five letters

**84** Regarding contrast sensitivity, which of the following statements are true and which are false?

   **i.** Contrast sensitivity can be tested with the Pelli-Robson chart
   **ii.** Contrast sensitivity is reduced in eyes with cataracts
   **iii.** Contrast sensitivity peaks at 2.5 spatial frequency cycles/degree of visual angle
   **iv.** Contrast sensitivity represents the visual system's sensitivity to light
   **v.** Contrast sensitivity can be tested with an Ishihara chart

**85** Regarding visual acuity (VA), which of the following statements are true and which are false?

   **i.** VA decreases with increased illuminance
   **ii.** VA decreases with increased duration of stimulus
   **iii.** VA decreases with increased size of stimulus
   **iv.** VA decreases with increased refractive error
   **v.** VA acuity decreases with increased retinal eccentricity

**86** Regarding colour vision, which of the following statements are true and which are false?

   **i.** Colour is perceived at the retinal level
   **ii.** The cones have maximum absorbance at 400, 540 and 700 nm
   **iii.** Blue cones are the most abundant
   **iv.** Rods are involved in colour vision
   **v.** Colour perceived is independent of illumination

**87** Regarding stereopsis, which of the following statements are true and which are false?

   **i.** Stereopsis is the ability to see an object in three dimensions
   **ii.** Is present at birth
   **iii.** Is fully developed by 4 months
   **iv.** Is poor beyond 20 degrees from the fovea
   **v.** Can be measured by the Lang test

**88** Regarding Panum's area, which of the following statements are true and which are false?

   **i.** It is the range of angular disparities over which vision is single and fused
   **ii.** Its area varies with the colour of the image
   **iii.** Its area varies with the size of the image
   **iv.** Its area varies with the eccentricity of the image
   **v.** Its area is larger in the horizontal meridian than the vertical meridian

89 Regarding the parvocellular pathway, which of the following statements are true and which are false?
   i. The parvocellular pathway conveys colour information
   ii. The parvocellular pathway has a faster response than the magnocellular pathway
   iii. The parvocellular pathway has a more rapid speed of conduction than the magnocellular pathway
   iv. The parvocellular pathway has smaller receptive fields than the magnocellular pathway
   v. The parvocelluar pathway is important for spatial discrimination

90 Regarding the magnocellular pathway, which of the following statements are true and which are false?
   i. The magnocelluar pathway is more responsive to moving targets than the parvocellular pathway
   ii. The magnocelluar pathway is more sensitive to light detection than the parvocellular pathway
   iii. The ganglia in the magnocellular pathway respond in a more transient way than the parvocellular pathway
   iv. The size of dendritic trees in the magnocellular pathway is larger than in the parvocellular pathway
   v. The magnocellular pathway exhibits linear spatial summation

91 Regarding optokinetic nystagmus, which of the following statements are true and which are false?
   i. It can be tested using a rotating drum
   ii. It is stimulated by the semicircular canals
   iii. It can be assessed using caloric testing
   iv. It is pathological
   v. It is a reflex

92 Regarding Horner's syndrome, which of the following statements are true and which are false?
   i. The ptosis only affects the upper lid
   ii. It is always associated with anhydrosis
   iii. Apraclonidine 0.5% drops may help in establishing a diagnosis of Horner's syndrome
   iv. Cocaine 4% drops may help in establishing the diagnosis of Horner's syndrome
   v. Hydroxyamphetamine 1% drops help to identify Horner's due to lesions of the third-order neurone

**93** Regarding Adie's tonic pupil, which of the following statements are true and which are false?
   i. It is always unilateral
   ii. Has a male predilection
   iii. There is slow constriction to prolonged near effort and slow redilation after near effort
   iv. There is absent or reduced light reaction
   v. It is a lesion of the sympathetic nervous system

**94** Regarding electroretinography (ERG), which of the following statements are true and which are false?
   i. The a-wave is produced by the retinal pigment epithelium
   ii. The b-wave is produced in the Müller cells
   iii. Full-field ERG is a measure of macula function
   iv. With the standard bright white flash, only a cone response is generated
   v. A 30-Hz flicker stimulus isolates the cone system

**95** Regarding the electro-oculogram (EOG), which of the following statements are true and which are false?
   i. EOG represents retinal pigment epithelial activity
   ii. EOG can distinguish between rod and cone dysfunction
   iii. EOG can distinguish between optic nerve and macula disease
   iv. If the EOG is abnormal, the ERG will always be abnormal
   v. The EOG is measured in dark adaptation followed by light adaptation

**96** Regarding visual evoked potentials (VEPs), which of the following statements are true and which are false?
   i. It is a measure of the response of the occipital cortex to visual stimulation
   ii. Pattern VEPs are elicited by a chequerboard pattern
   iii. In optic neuropathy, the VEPs show prolonged latency and decreased amplitude
   iv. It is not an appropriate test in children
   v. Latency is a more reliable indicator with VEPs than absolute amplitude

**97** Regarding dark adaptation, which of the following statements are true and which are false?

   i. Dark adaptation is the process by which the visual system adapts to decreased illumination

   ii. Dark adaptation curves form the basis of duplicity theory

   iii. The transition between rod- and cone-mediated vision is called the mesopic range

   iv. The time required for dark adaptation is dependent on the number of bleached rods

   v. Neural light adaptation is much faster than photochemical dark adaptation

**98** Regarding light-near dissociation, which of the following statements are true and which are false?

   i. The pupils demonstrate a better pupil response to light than near targets

   ii. It is found with Adie's pupil

   iii. It is found with Horner's syndrome

   iv. It is found with 6th nerve palsy

   v. It is found with a Marcus Gunn pupil

**99** Regarding Argyll Robertson pupils, which of the following statements are true and which are false?

   i. The pupils are small

   ii. The pupils do not dilate well with atropine

   iii. The pupils display light-near dissociation

   iv. The condition is usually bilateral

   v. Following cessation of the near target, the pupil response is tonic

**100** Regarding oxytocin, which of the following statements are true and which are false?

   i. It is released at the beginning of the menstrual cycle

   ii. It is structurally similar to vasopressin

   iii. It initiates contractions in the first stage of labour

   iv. It is structurally similar to aldosterone

   v. It initiates contractions in the second and third stages of labour

# 3

# Biochemistry and cell biology

# 30 FRCOphth best-fit MCQs

1  Which of the following statements regarding the ciliary body is least likely
   to be correct?
   a. It maintains the pressure of the eye via the secretion of aqueous
   b. Blood flow is under autonomic control
   c. The ciliary body secretes the main source of antioxidant systems in
      the anterior segment
   d. It forms part of the blood-retinal barrier

2  Which of the following structures has the highest lipid content?
   a. Retina
   b. Choroid
   c. Lens
   d. Cornea

3  Which of the following molecules is *not* thought to play a role in inter-
   retinal cell adhesion?
   a. Fibronectin
   b. ICAM-1
   c. CD44 antigen
   d. CD1 antigen

4  Which of the following statements regarding the cornea is *not* true?
   a. Hemidesmosomes are present on the corneal epithelial layer
   b. Fodrin and E-cadherin changes precede actin rearrangement
   c. Type II collagen is essential in the adhesion of corneal epithelium
      basement membrane to Bowman's layer
   d. Matrix metalloproteinases have been implicated in the repair of
      corneal epithelial defects

5  Which of the following mechanisms lowers intraocular pressure in the
   ciliary body?
   a. Stimulation of $\beta_2$ receptors through activation of adenylate cyclase
   b. Stimulation of $\alpha_2$ receptors through activation of adenylate cyclase
   c. Stimulation of $\alpha_2$ receptors through inhibition of adenylate cyclase
   d. Stimulation of $\beta_2$ receptors through inhibition of adenylate cyclase

6 Which of the following is *not* a physiological characteristic of trabecular meshwork cells?
  a. Low concentrations of microtubules
  b. Active phagocytic properties
  c. High concentrations of actin within their cytoplasm
  d. High concentrations of microtubules

7 Which of the following molecules is *not* required to form a G protein receptor?
  a. G protein
  b. Adenyl cyclase
  c. cCMP-dependent protein kinase
  d. cAMP-dependent protein kinase

8 Mitochondria:
  a. Are approximately 10 mm in size
  b. Consist of an inner core of sheets of cisternae
  c. Are a main site of storage of calcium
  d. Generate free radicals

9 Which of the following statements about endocytosis is *not* true?
  a. Primary lysosomes play an important role
  b. Clathrin-coated pits initially are on the cell surface
  c. Latrunculin B allows movement of the primary lysosome
  d. Once the vesicle is fully intracellular, it is known as an endosome

10 Which of the following statements is true about photoreceptors?
  a. Complete rod outer segment renewal takes around 21 days
  b. Photoreceptor turnover occurs in a diurnal manner
  c. Photoreceptors utilise glucose exclusively anaerobically
  d. Cone phagocytosis appears to occurs in a sequential manner

11 Which of the following statements is *true* regarding intercellular filaments and junctions?
  a. Gap junctions are highly organised and comprise ICAM-1 adhesions
  b. Desmosomes are approximately 40 nm in width
  c. The major protein present in tight junctions is occludin
  d. Synapse junctions occur in cartilage

**12** Which of the following cytokines is involved in eosinophil activation?
   **a.** IL-5
   **b.** IL-12
   **c.** IFN-γ
   **d.** GM-CSF

**13** Regarding DNA, which of the following statements is not true?
   **a.** Euchromatin is folded less tightly than heterochromatin
   **b.** The nucleolus contains fibrillar material and RNA
   **c.** Tightly folded chromatin in the nucleus permits transcription
   **d.** Basic proteins in the nucleus contain a positive charge

**14** Which of the following statements is *not true* regarding cytokines?
   **a.** They are effective only at very high concentrations
   **b.** They are short-term molecules
   **c.** They are secreted by cells in response to a specific stimulus
   **d.** They can stimulate secondary cytokine release

**15** Detoxification of free radicals occurs by:
   **a.** Vitamin B
   **b.** RNA polymerase
   **c.** Thymidylate kinase
   **d.** Catalase

**16** Arachidonic acid is derived from:
   **a.** Phospholipase $A_2$
   **b.** Thromboxane $A_2$
   **c.** $LTB_4$
   **d.** Prostaglandin $E_2$

**17** Which of the following is *not* mediated by the histamine type-1 receptor?
   **a.** CNS depression
   **b.** Smooth muscle contraction
   **c.** Increased vascular permeability
   **d.** Increased pepsin production

**18** A partial agonist:
   **a.** Has a high $EC_{50}$
   **b.** Exclusively prevents receptor activation
   **c.** Stimulates the receptor at a low concentration
   **d.** Possesses both agonist and antagonist properties

19  Which of the following techniques is best used to identify specific nucleic acid sequences?
   a. Flow cytometry
   b. In situ hybridisation
   c. Western blotting
   d. Northern blotting

20  Which of the following statements regarding lens metabolism is true?
   a. Increased degradation of MIP26 occurs with age
   b. Calpactins are not found in the lens
   c. Alpha-adrenergic compounds enhance the phosphorlyation of intermediate filaments
   d. Crystallins are restricted to the lens

21  Which of the following statements is *not* true regarding the vitreous gel?
   a. It is non-compressible
   b. It has a very high content of hyaluronic acid
   c. It promotes the bulk flow of fluid
   d. It behaves as a shock absorber

22  Which of the following statements is *not* true regarding the rough endoplasmic reticulum?
   a. It is studded with ribosomes
   b. It is arranged in rows within the cytoplasm
   c. Proteins are produced which are then folded within the internal elements of the structure
   d. It is the site of synthesis of steroids

23  The gel-like properties of the intracellular matrix are from:
   a. Microfilaments
   b. Rough endoplasmic reticulum
   c. Smooth endoplasmic reticulum
   d. Golgi apparatus

24  Which of the following is the most common side effect of the immunosuppressant cyclosporin?
   a. Hirsutism
   b. Osteoporosis
   c. Hypertension
   d. Nephrotoxicity

**25** Binding of epithelium to basement membrane is principally by:
  a. Adherens-type junctions
  b. Negative pressure
  c. Polarity
  d. Laminin

**26** Which of the following statements about immunohistochemistry is *not* true?
  a. Antigens can be preserved in a better way by exposure to microwaves
  b. It is very useful in the classification of malignant lymphoid cells
  c. The study of melanin is masked by the brown stain induced by the peroxidise-antiperoxidase reaction
  d. The technique is only used *in vivo*

**27** Which of the following statements about the choroid is *not* true?
  a. 98% of blood flow to the eye passes through the uveal tract
  b. The choroid has its own intrinsic lymphoid system
  c. There are large numbers of fenestrated capillaries
  d. Its oxygen consumption is very low compared to other tissues

**28** Which one of the following statements is true regarding retinal pigment epithelial cells?
  a. Turnover is rapid
  b. They express leucocyte marker CD40
  c. They possess GLUT-1 and -3 receptors
  d. They synthesise IL-2 regularly

**29** Regarding the blood-retinal barrier, which size of molecules are *not* able to pass through retinal vessels?
  a. 1000 Da
  b. 8000 Da
  c. 10 000 Da
  d. 20 000 Da

**30** Which of the following statements regarding the sclera is *not* true?
  a. Contractile filaments exist in the sclera
  b. The matrix is essentially acellular
  c. The sclera contains low concentrations of fibroblasts
  d. The distribution of collagen is highly irregular

# 30 ICO true/false MCQs

**31** Regarding diabetic ketoacidosis, which of the following statements are true and which are false?

   i. Metabolic acidosis results from a marked increase in ketones and amino acids

   ii. Hypovolemia results from an osmotic diuresis

   iii. Gluconeogenesis decreases liver output of glucose

   iv. Acetone smells from the breath are a result of increasing ketone concentration

   v. There is a decrease in lipolysis

**32** Regarding transcription factors, which of the following statements are true and which are false?

   i. NF-κB is a transciption factor

   ii. AP-1 is not a transcription factor

   iii. c-Jun is a transcription factor

   iv. GLUT-1 is not a transcription factor

   v. c-Fos is not a transcription factor

**33** Regarding the cell cycle, which of the following statements are true and which are false?

   i. S-phase chromosomal DNA is duplicated

   ii. Phase $G_2$ separates S phase from M phase

   iii. Chromosomes align along the equator of the cell in M phase

   iv. In a human fibroblast cell, the M phase lasts 10–12 hrs

   v. Cells in $G_0$ phase have a high metabolic rate

**34** Regarding intraocular pressure (IOP), which of the following statements are true and which are false?

   i. IOP is affected by circadian rhythms

   ii. IOP is affected by episcleral venous pressure

   iii. IOP is affected by anterior segment anatomy

   iv. IOP is affected by arterial pressure

   v. IOP is affected by hormonal influences

**35** Regarding haemoglobin, which of the following statements are true and which are false?

    **i.** An increase in carbon dioxide levels within the red cell decreases the affinity of haemoglobin for oxygen

    **ii.** Sickle-cell haemoglobin is more soluble than normal adult haemoglobin when oxygenated

    **iii.** It contains three atoms of iron which are in the FeII oxidation state

    **iv.** The polypeptide chains are linked by disulphide bonds

    **v.** Foetal human haemoglobin contains two alpha ($\alpha$) and two gamma ($\gamma$) units

**36** Regarding intracellular contents, which of the following statements are true and which are false?

    **i.** Membranes within mitochondria are folded to form cristae

    **ii.** Mitochondria act as a sodium store

    **iii.** Mitochondria have an abundance of histone proteins

    **iv.** Transmission of genetic mutations in mitochondria is purely paternal

    **v.** The aspartate/glutamate transport system is present within mitochondria

**37** Regarding energy production, which of the following statements are true and which are false?

    **i.** Pyruvate can be transaminated to lactate

    **ii.** Acetyl-CoA acts as a feedback propagator for pyruvate dehydrogenase

    **iii.** Pyruvate is generated from glucose

    **iv.** Dihydrolipoyl transacetylase is essential for the transfer of the acetyl group to coenzyme A

    **v.** Acetyl-CoA can be generated via $\beta$-oxidation from free fatty acids

**38** Regarding intracellular effects of hormones, which of the following statements are true and which are false?

    **i.** Secondary messengers commonly encountered in hormonal action are cyclic AMP and cyclic GMP

    **ii.** Inhibition of adenylate cyclase increases cyclic GMP levels which in turn activate protein kinase C

    **iii.** The effects of cyclic AMP are terminated when hydrolysed by phosphodiesterase

    **iv.** Transcription factors are inhibited by cyclic AMP

    **v.** Signal transduction often has an amplifying effect

**39** Regarding vitamins, which of the following statements are true and which are false?

    **i.** Vitamin A is water soluble

    **ii.** Tocopherol is also known as Vitamin E

    **iii.** Thiamine is fat soluble

    **iv.** Vitamin $B_{12}$ is synthesised by microorganisms

    **v.** Ascorbic acid is essential for the synthesis of collagen

**40** Regarding disorders of inborn metabolism, which of the following statements are true and which are false?

    **i.** Homocysteinuria is a disorder of tyrosine amino acid metabolism

    **ii.** Tyrosinaemia type I occurs due to a defect in the enzyme tyrosine aminotransferase

    **iii.** Albinism occurs due to a defect in the tyrosinase enzyme

    **iv.** Glucose 6-phosphatase deficiency principally affects the liver and kidney

    **v.** A defect in phenylalanine hydroxylase results in phenylketonuria

**41** Regarding glucose transport, which of the following statements are true and which are false?

    **i.** GLUT-1 transporter is not present in erythrocytes

    **ii.** GLUT-3 is present in the brain

    **iii.** GLUT-2 is present in high concentrations in the pancreas

    **iv.** Glucose is converted to fructose 1,6-bisphosphate in the last step of glycolysis

    **v.** GLUT-5 is important for fructose absorption

**42** Regarding tissue proteins, which of the following statements are true and which are false?

    **i.** Collagen type II is present in the stroma

    **ii.** Aggrecan is present in tissue cartilage

    **iii.** Thrombospondins are present within lymphocytes

    **iv.** Tissue inhibitors of metalloproteinases (TIMPs) are involved in tissue remodelling

    **v.** Fibrillin is found in the lens

**43** Regarding mitochondria, which of the following statements are true and which are false?

   i. They are usually 1 µm in diameter
   ii. The internal matrix is known as the mitosol
   iii. They generate approximately 60% of the ATP required by the cell
   iv. Cytochrome d plays an essential role in apoptosis
   v. They play a role in their own replication

**44** Regarding nuclei, which of the following statements are true and which are false?

   i. Chromatin consists of DNA only
   ii. Chromatin consists of DNA and RNA only
   iii. Euchromatin is more densely packed than heterochromatin
   iv. The nucleolus is the site of ribosomal RNA synthesis
   v. The rough endoplasmic reticulum is the site of ribosomal RNA synthesis

**45** Regarding lysosomes, which of the following statements are true and which are false?

   i. They maintain an alkaline pH of 8
   ii. They can act through endocytosis
   iii. They contain the enzyme collagenase
   iv. They do not contain the enzyme hyaluronidase
   v. They are not involved in autophagy

**46** Regarding the cornea, which of the following statements are true and which are false?

   i. Type IV and VII collagen are present
   ii. Epithelial cells express laminin and collagen
   iii. Hemidesmosomes are absent
   iv. Cells are adherent via zonula occludens
   v. Stromal collagen is predominantly type 2

**47** Regarding the ciliary body, which of the following statements are true and which are false?

   i. It contains a low concentration of hyalase
   ii. Glutathione peroxidise is important in the detoxification of peroxides
   iii. Hydrogen peroxide is a byproduct and is excreted by the cornea
   iv. Melatonin helps remove hydrogen peroxide
   v. Prostaglandin formation is suppressed by the ciliary body during inflammation

**48** Regarding the lens, which of the following statements are true and which are false?

    **i.** Crystallins make up 90% of lens protein

    **ii.** β-crystallins trap other proteins and filaments

    **iii.** The microfilament vimentin is absent in the lens in vivo

    **iv.** Cytokeratins are not found in the adult lens

    **v.** The lens capsule contains type IV collagen

**49** Regarding the vitreous, which of the following statements are true and which are false?

    **i.** The vitreous is 70% water

    **ii.** The spaces between collagen fibrils are filled with glycosaminoglycans (GAGs)

    **iii.** Hyaluronic acid increases in concentration with age

    **iv.** Type VI collagen is absent

    **v.** Hyalocytes produce hyaluronic acid

**50** Regarding the following peptides, which of the following statements are true and which are false?

    **i.** Glutamate acts on photoreceptors

    **ii.** Serotonin acts on photoreceptors

    **iii.** Substance P acts on amacrine and ganglion cells

    **iv.** Neurotensin acts on amacrine cells

    **v.** β-endorphin acts on photoreceptor cells

**51** Regarding aqueous secretion, which of the following statements are true and which are false?

    **i.** Adrenergic agonists are absent in the iris

    **ii.** Muscarinic receptors are absent in the ciliary body

    **iii.** The majority of the receptors in the ciliary body are β1

    **iv.** Blockage of β2 receptors leads to an increase in aqueous secretion

    **v.** Adrenergic receptors are present in the ciliary body

**52** Regarding cell membranes, which of the following statements are true and which are false?

    **i.** The cell membrane separates the cytoplasm from the external environment

    **ii.** The cell membrane is made up of lipids principally

    **iii.** The cell membrane is made up of glucose principally

    **iv.** Cell membranes are involved in cell signalling

    **v.** Cell membranes are involved in cell-to-cell adhesion

53 Regarding the Krebs cycle, which of the following statements are true and which are false?
  i. Succinyl CoA is an essential component
  ii. Pyruvate is a non-essential component
  iii. Three ATP molecules are generated per turn of the cycle
  iv. The regulation of the Krebs cycle is partly due to substrate availability
  v. Pyruvate is used for feedback inhibition

54 Regarding vascular endothelial growth factor (VEGF), which of the following statements are true and which are false?
  i. It stimulates angiogenesis
  ii. It inhibits neovascularisation
  iii. Bevacizumab inhibits VEGF
  iv. It decreases the mitotic rate of endothelial cells
  v. It is upregulated by hypoxia inducible factor (HIF)

55 Regarding vitamin A, which of the following statements are true and which are false?
  i. Vitamin A is required for epithelial keratin expression
  ii. Vitamin A is required for vimentin expression
  iii. Vitamin A is essential for corneal wound healing
  iv. Vitamin A is essential to inhibit proteolytic enzymes
  v. Vitamin A deficiency results in Bitot's spots

56 Regarding cataract formation, which of the following statements are true and which are false?
  i. There is increased cytoskeletal organisation of cells
  ii. There is an increase in enzymatic activity in the lens
  iii. Production of β-crystallin increases with age
  iv. There is an increase in water content with age
  v. The lens contains a high concentration of glutathione

57 Regarding the blood-retinal barrier, which of the following statements are true and which are false?
  i. It is maintained by tight junctions
  ii. Retinal vessels are impermeable to molecules larger than 100 000 Da
  iii. Nitric oxide constricts retinal vasculature
  iv. Pericytes possess contractile properties that regulate blood flow
  v. Pericytes possess high levels of IGF-1 and IGF-2

**58** Regarding the retina, which of the following statements are true and which are false?

  i. There is a continuous turnover of rod outer segments
  ii. Tunicamycin inhibits the glycosylation of rhodopsin
  iii. Rod outer segment disc shedding occurs in a diurnal manner
  iv. Phagocytosis of the disc outer segment occurs in the retinal pigment epithelium (RPE)
  v. There is rapid turnover of cone outer segments

**59** Regarding retinal transduction, which of the following statements are true and which are false?

  i. Rhodopsin is activated via the isomerisation of retinol
  ii. All-trans-retinal inserts into the rhodopsin transmembrane loops
  iii. Cellular retinal binding protein is present in the disc outer segment
  iv. Vitamin A deficiency initially results in visual deterioration in high levels of illumination
  v. An amplification cascade ensures a large amount of energy is released per photon of light

**60** Regarding neurotransmitters in the retina, which of the following statements are true and which are false?

  i. GABA is an inhibitory transmitter
  ii. Glycine is an excitatory transmitter
  iii. L-aspartate is an excitatory transmitter
  iv. Acetylcholine is an excitatory transmitter
  v. Dopamine is an inhibitory transmitter

# 4
# Pathology

# 30 FRCOphth best-fit MCQs

1   Oil Red O is a stain that is used for:
    a. Lipid
    b. Mucopolysaccharide
    c. Descemet's membrane
    d. Mucin

2   The following is an example of physiological hyperplasia:
    a. Prostate enlargement in older age
    b. Breast enlargement during puberty
    c. Uterine growth during pregnancy
    d. Thyroid enlargement due to excessive TSH

3   Which of the following does *not* predispose a patient to thrombosis?
    a. Lupus anticoagulant
    b. Antithrombin III deficiency
    c. Hypoviscosity
    d. Protein C deficiency

4   Basal cell carcinomas are commonly seen in:
    a. Fitz-Hugh and Curtis syndrome
    b. Gorlin-Goltz syndrome
    c. Hermansky-Pudlak syndrome
    d. Chédiak-Higashi syndrome

5   Which of the following are *not* recognized chemical mediators of inflammation?
    a. Prostaglandin E
    b. Dopamine
    c. TNF-α
    d. Bradykinin

6   Which of the following conditions are *not* associated with amyloid deposition?
    a. Alzheimer's disease
    b. Haemodialysis associated
    c. Familial Mediterranean fever
    d. Gaucher's disease

**7** A mother with no family history of retinoblastoma has a child with unilateral retinoblastoma – what is the risk of a second child having the condition?
   **a.** 1%
   **b.** 33%
   **c.** 40%
   **d.** 50%

**8** Regarding age-related macular degeneration, drusen are located:
   **a.** Between the outer nuclear layer and photoreceptor layer
   **b.** Between the photoreceptor layer and retinal pigment epithelium
   **c.** Between the retinal pigment epithelium and Bruch's membrane
   **d.** Between Bruch's membrane and the choroid

**9** The following is *not* a feature of choroidal melanomas:
   **a.** Collar studding
   **b.** Spindle C cells
   **c.** Epithelioid cells
   **d.** Subretinal fluid

**10** Which of the following is *not* a recognized oncogene?
   **a.** *Ras*
   **b.** *Myc*
   **c.** *p53*
   **d.** *Abl*

**11** Optic nerve glioma are associated with:
   **a.** Neurofibromatosis type 1
   **b.** Sturge-Weber syndrome
   **c.** Tuberous sclerosis
   **d.** Von Hippel-Lindau syndrome

**12** Atherosclerosis is *not* characterised by:
   **a.** Infiltration of mononuclear leucocytes
   **b.** Release of platelet-derived growth factor
   **c.** Increased nitric oxide : acetylcholine ratio
   **d.** Proliferation of smooth muscle cells

**13** A typical 'Swiss cheese' histological appearance is pathognomonic of:
   **a.** Lacrimal gland pleomorphic adenoma
   **b.** Dacroadenitis
   **c.** Lacrimal gland adenoid cystic carcinoma
   **d.** Sarcoidosis

**14** Which of the following types of retinal embolus may also be called a Hollenhorst plaque?
   a. Cholesterol
   b. Platelet
   c. Thrombus
   d. Bacteria

**15** Immune complex-mediated (type III) hypersensitivity:
   a. Is mediated by T-cells
   b. Leads to granulomatous inflammation
   c. Is seen in ocular cicatricial pemphygoid
   d. Is seen in systemic lupus erythematosus

**16** Regarding apoptosis:
   a. Chromatin condensation and DNA fragmentation are seen
   b. Cell membrane integrity is lost
   c. There is an associated inflammatory response
   d. Lytic enzymes are released from lysosomes

**17** Which of the following is *not* a consequence of ATP depletion in hypoxia?
   a. Failure of ATP-dependent sodium and potassium pumps causing cell swelling
   b. Increased anaerobic glycolysis
   c. Increase in intracellular pH
   d. Reduced protein synthesis

**18** Which of the following is *not* a feature of hyperacute graft rejection?
   a. Presence of circulating antibodies to graft antigens
   b. Intimal fibrosis
   c. Occurs within minutes
   d. Complement activation

**19** A corneal specimen from a patient with Avellino dystrophy would stain with the following:
   a. Masson trichrome and Alcian blue
   b. Congo red and Masson trichrome
   c. Congo red and Alcian blue
   d. Congo red and Alizarin red

**20** Which of the following corneal abnormalities would *not* stain with Prussian blue?
   **a.** Fleischer ring
   **b.** Vogt's striae
   **c.** Stocker line
   **d.** Ferry line

**21** Histological associations of diabetic retinopathy do *not* include:
   **a.** Selective loss of pericytes
   **b.** Deposition of amyloid
   **c.** Thickening of the retinal capillary basement membrane
   **d.** Retinal capillary closure

**22** Touton giant cells are commonly found in:
   **a.** Giant cell arteritis
   **b.** Tuberculosis
   **c.** Juvenile xanthogranuloma
   **d.** Sarcoidosis

**23** Which of the following is not a feature of Fuchs' endothelial dystrophy?
   **a.** Sparse endothelial cells
   **b.** Epithelial microcysts
   **c.** Excrescences of Bowman's membrane
   **d.** 'Beaten bronze' appearance

**24** Benign tumours are characterised by which of the following?
   **a.** Ability to metastasise
   **b.** Well differentiated
   **c.** Nuclear pleomorphism
   **d.** Increased number of nuclear mitotic figures

**25** Which of the following viruses is *not* associated with tumour formation?
   **a.** Epstein-Barr virus
   **b.** Hepatitis B virus
   **c.** Hepatitis A virus
   **d.** Human immunodeficiency virus

**26** What is the most common cause of septic shock?
   **a.** Gram-positive bacilli expressing exotoxin
   **b.** Gram-positive bacilli expressing endotoxin
   **c.** Gram-negative bacilli expressing exotoxin
   **d.** Gram-negative bacilli expressing endotoxin

27 Which of the following is true in wound healing by primary intention?
   a. It is less common than healing by secondary intention
   b. The wound is not sutured
   c. Healing is faster than that by secondary intention
   d. Healing is largely by granulation

28 Which of the following definitions is correct?
   a. Hyperplasia is an increase in cell size without cell division
   b. Hypertrophy is an increase in cell number by mitosis
   c. Metaplasia is a reversible transformation of one undifferentiated cell type into another undifferentiated cell type
   d. Dysplasia is increased cell growth with atypia and decreased differentiation

29 Which of the following is involved in promoting angiogenesis?
   a. Serotonin
   b. Interferon-alpha
   c. Matrix metalloproteinases
   d. Thrombospondin

30 Keratin pearls are commonly seen in:
   a. Merkel cell carcinoma
   b. Basal cell carcinoma
   c. Squamous cell carcinoma
   d. Sebaceous cell carcinoma

# 30 ICO true/false MCQs

**31** Concerning intracranial meningiomas, which of the following are true and which are false?

   i. A common clinical sign is optic nerve pallor

   ii. Meningiomas that arise from the olfactory groove or the sphenoid cause a 7th (facial) nerve palsy, a false localising sign

   iii. Psammoma bodies are a common pathological finding

   iv. A common finding is type A spindle cells

   v. A common finding is IgM in cell cytoplasm

**32** Concerning giant cell arteritis, which of the following are true and which are false?

   i. Inflammatory cells are often present in the internal elastic lamina

   ii. Multinucleate cells are often absent

   iii. Haematoxylin and eosin stain is often used

   iv. Tongue claudication is a pathognomonic clinical sign

   v. 35% of cases have a normal ESR and CRP

**33** Regarding pterygia, which of the following are true and which are false?

   i. Stromal elastosis is classical

   ii. Inheritance is autosomal dominant

   iii. Eosinophils predominate basophils

   iv. Beta radiation is commonly used

   v. Cystic spaces are more common in naevi

**34** Regarding stains in histopathology, which of the following are true and which are false?

   i. Haematoxylin and eosin stains nuclei and ribosomes

   ii. Periodic acid-Schiff stains viruses

   iii. Giemsa helps identify chlamydia

   iv. Ziehl–Neelsen is used in tuberculosis detection

   v. Gram staining is useful in *Acanthamoeba* detection

**35** Regarding wound healing, which of the following are true and which are false?
  i. The proliferation phase is characterised by angiogenesis
  ii. Fibronectin is essential in extracellular matrix formation
  iii. Interleukin 7 is a neutrophil chemoattractant
  iv. The growth factor transforming growth factor beta (TGF-β) stimulates proliferation
  v. Primary intention involves breach of the dermis

**36** Regarding tissue stains, which of the following are true and which are false?
  i. Alcian blue stains mucopolysaccharide
  ii. Colloidal iron stains calcium
  iii. Congo red is useful in staining amyloid
  iv. Oil Red O and Prussian blue help identify iron
  v. Alizarin red is useful in macular corneal dystrophy

**37** Regarding hypertrophy, which of the following are true and which are false?
  i. It involves an increase in cell size
  ii. It involves an increase in cell number
  iii. It commonly occurs in cardiac muscle
  iv. It commonly occurs in the liver
  v. It commonly occurs in skeletal muscle

**38** In macular corneal dystrophy, which of the following statements are true and which are false?
  i. Alcian blue can be useful in the histopathological diagnosis
  ii. Prussian blue can be useful in the diagnosis
  iii. Staining of mucopolysaccharide is evident
  iv. The inheritance is mitochondrial
  v. The inheritance is autosomal recessive

**39** Regarding metastatic tumours, which of the following statements are true and which are false?
  i. They can spread through the lymphatic system
  ii. Actin and myosin are often expressed
  iii. The breast is the most common site for tumours to metastasise
  iv. Metastases increase osteoclastic activity
  v. They show a decrease in glucose transport

**40** Regarding choroidal melanomas, which of the following statements are true and which are false?
  i. They typically contain plump nuclei
  ii. They can contain spindle C cells
  iii. Epitheloid cells have oval nuclei
  iv. A 'collar stud' appearance is often evident in choroidal melanomas
  v. Choroidal melanomas with a predominantly epitheloid cell type have the worst prognosis

**41** Regarding vascular leakage, which of the following statements are true and which are false?
  i. It results from endothelial contraction
  ii. It may result from direct injury
  iii. It is a hallmark of chronic inflammation
  iv. Protein-rich fluid is retained within the blood vessel
  v. It is dependent on an increased hydrostatic pressure in the vessel

**42** Regarding metaplasia, which of the following statements are true and which are false?
  i. Metaplasia is irreversible
  ii. The most common adaptive metaplasia is squamous cell metaplasia in the human lung
  iii. Vitamin B deficiency induces squamous metaplasia of the respiratory epithelium
  iv. It never occurs in mesenchymal cells
  v. Controlling metaplasia is one principle behind stem cell research

**43** Regarding cell injury, which of the following statements are true and which are false?
  i. Nuclear chromatin is prominent
  ii. Nuclear material undergoes fragmentation
  iii. Liquefactive necrosis occurs in myocardial infarction
  iv. Caseous necrosis is often present in tuberculosis infection
  v. Enzymatic fat necrosis has been observed in the pancreas

**44** Regarding melanosis of the conjunctiva, which of the following statements are true and which are false?

 i. Racial melanosis tends to be bilateral and symmetrical
 ii. Primary acquired melanosis without atypia rarely progresses to melanoma
 iii. The smaller the area of primary acquired melanosis with atypia, the greater the chance of progression to conjunctival melanoma
 iv. 20% of conjunctival melanomas arise de novo
 v. Conjunctival melanomas tend to present in the fifth to sixth decade of life

**45** Regarding the vasculitides, which of the following are true and which are false?

 i. Antineutrophil anticytoplasmic antibodies are present in Wegener's granulomatosis
 ii. p-ANCA are directed towards myeloperoxidase
 iii. Antiendothelial antibodies are present in giant cell (temporal) arteritis
 iv. Anti-DNA immune complexes are observed in Takayasu's arteritis
 v. Syphilis, a fungus, can induce an infectious vasculitis

**46** Regarding corneal dystrophies, which of the following statements are true and which are false?

 i. Lattice dystrophy is an epithelial dystrophy
 ii. Macular dystrophy is an autosomal dominant disorder
 iii. Hyaline bodies and keratinoid (keratin-like substance) are features of granular dystrophy
 iv. Labrador keratopathy is often present in patients with chronic sun exposure
 v. Hassall-Henle warts are features of posterior polymorphous endothelial dystrophy

**47** Regarding diabetic eye disease, which of the following statements are true and which are false?

 i. Proliferative diabetic retinopathy features the growth of new vessels
 ii. Cranial nerve palsies can occur, which affect the extraocular muscles
 iii. Diabetic patients are more prone to posterior subcapsular cataracts
 iv. The corneal epithelium heals poorly
 v. Clinically significant diabetic macular oedema is highly responsive to treatment

**48** Regarding amino acid metabolism, which of the following statements are true and which are false?
  i. Homocystinuria is characterised by an increase in the levels of cystathionine β-synthetase
  ii. Homocystinuria is characterised by the inferonasal dislocation of the natural lens
  iii. Homocystinuria is characterised by an increased susceptibility to thrombus formation
  iv. Cystinosis is characterised by the accumulation of cystine crystals in the conjunctiva, cornea, choroid and retina
  v. Cystinosis is characterised by accumulation of cystine within lysosomes

**49** Regarding the phakomatoses, which of the following statements are true and which are false?
  i. Neurofibromatosis is an autosomal dominant condition
  ii. Lisch nodules consist of melanocytic proliferations on the anterior surface of the iris
  iii. Optic nerve gliomas never occur
  iv. Astrocytic hamartomas form within the retina in tuberous sclerosis
  v. Sturge-Weber syndrome is inherited in an autosomal recessive pattern

**50** Regarding techniques in pathology, which of the following statements are true and which are false?
  i. Flow cytometry is a technique used to isolate genotype specific cells
  ii. Avidin biotin is useful for paraffin sections
  iii. Proliferative activity can be measured using Ki67
  iv. Impression cytology is useful in the assessment of conjunctival diseases
  v. Haematoxylin and eosin are the most commonly used stains in histopathology

**51** Regarding thyroid eye disease, which of the following statements are true and which are false?
  i. Exophthalmos is never unilateral
  ii. $T_3$ and $T_4$ levels are usually high in hyperthyroidism
  iii. Extraocular muscle tendons are usually swollen on magnetic resonance imaging
  iv. Perivascular lymphocytic infiltration is usually visible on histological examination
  v. Loss of sensory nerves results in external ophthalmoplegia

**52** Regarding retinal haemorrhages, which of the following statements are true and which are false?
   i. Dot haemorrhages result from a rupture of capillaries in the internal limiting membrane
   ii. Flame haemorrhages consist of haemorrhage tracking in the nerve fibre layer
   iii. Blot haemorrhages result from capillary haemorrhages into the retrohyaloid space
   iv. Intraretinal microvascular anomalies represent growth into the vitreous
   v. Vitreous haemorrhage never occurs in retinopathy of prematurity

**53** Regarding reversible cell injury, which of the following statements are true and which are false?
   i. Autophagy of lysosomes occurs
   ii. Endoplasmic reticulum lysis occurs
   iii. Bleb formation of cell membranes occurs
   iv. Nuclear pyknosis and karyolyis occurs
   v. Mitochondial swelling occurs

**54** Regarding chemical mediators of inflammation, which of the following statements are true and which are false?
   i. Thromboxane $A_2$ is involved in vasodilation
   ii. Leukotriene $B_4$ is involved in chemotaxis
   iii. Prostanglandin $E_2$ is involved in inflammatory vasodilation
   iv. Thromboxane $A_2$ is a potent platelet aggregator
   v. Platelet activating factor is derived from mast cells

**55** Regarding interleukin 1, which of the following statements are true and which are false?
   i. IL-1 induces an increase in fever
   ii. IL-1 increases leucocyte adherence
   iii. IL-1 increases procoagulant activity
   iv. IL-1increases fibroblastic activity
   v. IL-1 increases prostaglandin activity

**56** Regarding fibroblast growth factor (FGF), which of the following statements are true and which are false?

i. FGF induces monocyte chemotaxis

ii. FGF induces fibroblast migration

iii. FGF induces fibroblast proliferation

iv. FGF induces collagenase secretion

v. FGF induces angiogenesis

**57** Regarding basal cell carcinomas, which of the following statements are true and which are false?

i. They commonly occur in Gorlin-Goltz syndrome

ii. At the periphery, cells are arranged in a palisading pattern

iii. Ulceration in these tumours does not induce an inflammatory reaction

iv. Morphoeic basal cell carcinomas induce a strong fibroblastic reaction

v. They often have well-defined edges

**58** Regarding conjunctival melanomas, which of the following statements are true and which are false?

i. Caruncular or palpebral placement carries a better prognosis

ii. Mortality is 10% at 5 years

iii. Common sites for metastases include the kidneys

iv. Topical mitomycin C has been very effective in preventing local recurrence

v. Amelanotic melanomas are usually blue in colour

**59** Regarding Grocott's hexamine, which of the following statements are true and which are false?

i. It is used to stain parasites

ii. It is used to stain Gram-negative bacteria

iii. It is only used to stain lipopolysaccharide endotoxin

iv. It is used to stain spirochetes

v. It is used to stain fungi

**60** Regarding sarcoidosis, which of the following statements are true and which are false?

i. It frequently causes an increase in vitamin D production outside the kidney

ii. It involves a caseating granulomatous reaction

iii. It can present as lesions on the iris known as Lisch nodules

iv. Serum ACE is often a useful indicator

v. It can result in a multifocal choroiditis

# 5

# Microbiology and immunology

# 20 FRCOphth best-fit MCQs

**1** Which one of the following is eukaryotic?
   a. Bacteria
   b. *Rickettsia*
   c. *Chlamydia*
   d. *Candida*

**2** Which of the following does *not* increase bacterial virulence?
   a. Presence of pathogenicity islands in *Shigella*
   b. Presence of fibrillae in Gram-positive bacteria
   c. Endotoxins produced by Gram-positive bacteria
   d. Inhibition of lysosomal digestion by mycobacteria

**3** Which one of the following is true?
   a. Staphylococci are Gram-negative cocci
   b. Clostridia are Gram-negative bacilli
   c. *Neisseria* are Gram-negative cocci
   d. *Pseudomonas* are Gram-positive bacilli

**4** Which of the following organisms is a commensal found on the conjunctival surface?
   a. *Neisseria gonorrhoeae*
   b. *Streptococcus viridans*
   c. *Streptococcus pneumoniae*
   d. *Haemophilus influenzae*

**5** Which of the following is an RNA virus?
   a. Herpes simplex virus
   b. Cytomegalovirus
   c. Adenovirus
   d. Measles virus

**6** Which of the following is true regarding aciclovir?
   a. It acts via inhibiting viral DNA polymerase
   b. It is particularly effective in treating cytomegalovirus infection
   c. Oral use can cause renal dysfunction
   d. It is broken down slowly by infected host cells

7 Which one of the following is true regarding human immunodeficiency virus (HIV)?
   a. It is a DNA retrovirus
   b. It is clinically most commonly detected by PCR testing
   c. It leads to a diagnosis of AIDS when the CD4 count is less than 400
   d. It is associated with HHV-8 infection

8 Which of the following is *not* a risk factor for the development of fungal keratitis?
   a. Trauma with plant matter
   b. Vertical transmission
   c. Diabetes
   d. Hydrophilic contact lenses

9 Which of the following is true regarding *Acanthamoeba*?
   a. It is a type of *Rickettsia*
   b. It can be stained with periodic acid-Schiff stain
   c. It can be cultured on blood agar
   d. It is sensitive to topical amphotericin

10 Regarding sterilisation of instruments, autoclaves:
   a. Use dry heat
   b. Are effective in destroying bacterial spores
   c. Cannot be used for sterilising rubber
   d. Are used commercially for sterilising prepacked disposable instruments

11 Aminoglycosides:
   a. Are effective in treating *Escherichia coli*
   b. Interfere with bacterial cell wall synthesis
   c. Penetrate the blood-brain barrier
   d. Are bacteriostatic

12 Ciprofloxacin:
   a. Acts by inhibiting DNA gyrase
   b. Has a 10% cross-reactivity in patients allergic to cephalosporins
   c. Is effective only in treating Gram-negative bacterial infection
   d. Has poor ocular penetration

13 Which of the following is *not* a component of the innate immune system?
   a. Lysozyme in tears
   b. Macrophages
   c. Cytotoxic T-cells
   d. Complement

14 Which of the following is true regarding immunoglobulins?
   a. Immunoglobulin type is determined by the Fab region
   b. The Fc region recognises foreign material
   c. The heavy chain consists of V, C and D regions
   d. Antibody diversity is generated by rearrangement of the V, C and
      J immunoglobulin gene loci

15 Regarding mucosa-associated lymphoid tissue (MALT):
   a. It is not present in conjunctiva
   b. MALT is well encapsulated
   c. The predominant immunoglobulin produced is IgA
   d. Rarely, adenocarcinoma associated with this tissue may develop

16 Which type of hypersensitivity response is seen in ocular cicatricial
   pemphygoid?
   a. Type I
   b. Type II
   c. Type III
   d. Type IV

17 Regarding interferons:
   a. Interferon-α has antibacterial effects
   b. Interferon-α is produced by fibroblasts
   c. Interferon-β is mainly produced by leucocytes
   d. Interferon-β may be used in the treatment of multiple sclerosis

18 Regarding the major histocompatibility complex (MHC):
   a. It is an area on chromosome 12
   b. Class I encodes HLA antigens DR, DP, etc.
   c. Class I are expressed on virtually all nucleated cells
   d. Class I expression protects cells from destruction by cytotoxic T-cells

19  Which of the following is true regarding acute graft rejection?
   a.  It is predominantly antibody mediated
   b.  It is predominantly cell mediated
   c.  Corneal graft rejection is an example of type 2 hypersensitivity
   d.  HLA class II matching is routinely performed in corneal transplantation

20  Which of the following is true regarding complement?
   a.  Opsonisation is mediated by component C1q
   b.  Components C5–C9 form the membrane attack complex
   c.  The classical pathway is initiated by the cell walls of Gram-negative bacteria
   d.  The alternative pathway is activated in systemic lupus erythematosus

# 20 ICO true/false MCQs

**21** Regarding bacterial toxins, which of the following statements are true and which are false?
   i. Exotoxins may be produced by Gram-positive or Gram-negative bacteria
   ii. Endotoxins may be produced by Gram-positive or Gram-negative bacteria
   iii. Botulinum toxin is an example of an exotoxin
   iv. Superantigens are a group of exotoxins
   v. Endotoxins consist of peptidoglycan from the bacterial cell wall

**22** Regarding *Pseudomonas* species, which of the following statements are true and which are false?
   i. They are anaerobic Gram-negative rods
   ii. They possess flagella and pili improving adherence to host cells
   iii. They are able to penetrate an intact corneal epithelium
   iv. They can be cultured on blood agar
   iv. They are the commonest cause of contact lens-related corneal ulcers

**23** Regarding *Chlamydia* species, which of the following statements are true and which are false?
   i. They are able to replicate in the extracellular state
   ii. *Chlamydia trachomatis* serotypes D–K cause trachoma
   iii. *Chlamydia pneumoniae* serotypes A–C cause oculogenital disease
   iv. *Chlamydia* infection may present with chronic conjunctivitis
   v. Polymerase chain reaction (PCR) is the diagnostic investigation of choice

**24** Regarding the steps of viral replication, which of the following statements are true and which are false?
   i. Tissue tropism is determined by host cell surface receptors
   ii. Viral uptake is mediated by exocytosis
   iii. DNA viruses use the host cell DNA polymerase for transcription
   iv. RNA viruses encode their own RNA-dependent RNA polymerases
   v. Cell lysis is always necessary for release of viruses from the host cell

**25** Regarding herpes viruses, which of the following statements are true and which are false?

   i. They are double-stranded DNA viruses

   ii. Herpes simplex is able to establish latency in epithelial cells

   iii. Herpes zoster often causes dendritic ulceration of the cornea

   iv. Herpes simplex virus may cause retinal necrosis in immunocompetent patients

   v. Diagnosis is most commonly made using serology

**26** Regarding antiviral agents:

   i. Ganciclovir has better efficacy than aciclovir in the treatment for *Cytomegalovirus* infections

   ii. Nephrotoxicity is the main side effect of ganciclovir

   iii. Ganciclovir may be given orally

   iv. Foscarnet may be given via intravitreal injection

   v. Aciclovir is only toxic to cells infected by virus

**27** Regarding prions:

   i. They possess a genome but no envelope or capsid

   ii. They induce a marked inflammatory response

   iii. They may be destroyed by ionising radiation

   iv. They may be destroyed by autoclaving

   v. PCR is the diagnostic test of choice

**28** Which of the following statements regarding HIV are true and which are false?

   i. HIV binds to the CD8 receptor on the cell

   ii. The co-receptor for HIV is CCR5

   iii. HIV infects T-cells only

   iv. Reverse transcriptase encoded by HIV is highly reliable

   v. Viral DNA integrated into the host genome is termed provirus

**29** Regarding *Candida* infection, which of the following statements are true and which are false?

   i. It consists of tubular structures called hyphae

   ii. It is usually pathogenic

   iii. It is a common cause of exogenous endophthalmitis

   iv. It can be stained with calcofluor white

   v. Oral candidiasis is an AIDS-defining illness

**30** Regarding toxoplasmosis:
    i. It is an obligate intracellular parasite
    ii. The reservoir host is the dog
    iii. Infection occurs via aerosol transmission
    iv. Dragging of the optic disc may be seen
    v. Recurrent disease may occur

**31** Regarding penicillins, which of the following statements are true and which are false?
    i. They interfere with bacterial cell wall lipopolysaccharide synthesis
    ii. Benzylpenicillin is poorly absorbed in the gastrointestinal tract
    iii. Amoxicillin is effective in treating *Staphylococcus aureus* infections
    iv. Clavulanic acid aids bacterial cell wall permeability by the drug
    v. Penicillins are excreted by the kidney

**32** Regarding antifungal drugs:
    i. Amphotericin binds to ergosterol in fungal cell membranes
    ii. Amphotericin may be injected intravitreally to treat *Candida* endophthalmitis
    iii. Liver function tests must be monitored when intravenous amphotericin is administered
    iv. Fluconazole shows good central nervous system penetration
    v. Fluconazole may be administered orally

**33** Regarding syphilis infection, which of the following statements are true and which are false?
    i. It is caused by a Gram-positive bacillus
    ii. The causative agent can survive for several days outside the body
    iii. Argyll Robertson pupil may be a feature
    iv. Interstitial keratitis may be a feature
    v. Treatment is with high-dose penicillin

**34** Regarding classes of immunoglobulin, which of the following statements are true and which are false?
    i. IgG is able to fix complement via the C1 pathway
    ii. IgA is present in secretions from mucous membranes
    iii. IgM is produced late in the immune response
    iv. IgD is present on neutrophils
    v. IgE is bound to mast cells

**35** Which of the following is a role of the complement system?
   **i.** Chemotaxis
   **ii.** Opsonisation
   **iii.** Cytolysis
   **iv.** T-cell activation
   **v.** Antibody fixation

**36** Regarding antigen presentation, which of the following statements are true and which are false?
   **i.** T-cells are able to recognise free antigen
   **ii.** MHC class I binds endogenously synthesised antigen
   **iii.** MHC class II binds exogenously synthesised antigen
   **iv.** B-cells may be antigen-presenting cells
   **v.** Macrophages may present antigen bound to MHC class I molecules

**37** Which of the following are components of the ocular surface defences?
   **i.** Lysozyme
   **ii.** Complement
   **iii.** Polymorphonuclear leucocytes
   **iv.** IgM
   **v.** Cytotoxic T-cells

**38** Regarding treatment of uveitis, which of the following statements are true and which are false?
   **i.** Infliximab is an inhibitor of TNF-$\beta$
   **ii.** Adalimumab is an inhibitor of TNF-$\alpha$
   **iii.** TNF-$\alpha$ is produced by T-helper cells
   **iv.** Infliximab therapy may cause reactivation of tuberculosis
   **v.** Infliximab is not effective in treating HLA-B27 associated uveitis

**39** Regarding autoantibodies:
   **i.** Positive p-ANCA antibodies are associated with Wegener's granulomatosis
   **ii.** Anti-Ro and La antibodies are associated with Sjögren's syndrome
   **iii.** Anti-TSH receptor antibodies are associated with Hashimoto's thyroiditis
   **iv.** Anti-acetylcholine receptor antibodies are associated with myasthenia gravis
   **v.** Anti-double-stranded DNA antibodies are associated with ocular cicatricial pemphigoid

**40** Regarding the cytokines, which of the statements are true and which are false?
   i. Cytokines act in a paracrine manner
   ii. Cytokines have a long time course of action
   iii. Each cytokine has a specific effect
   iv. IL-1 is produced by macrophages
   v. TNF-α is produced by T-helper cells

# 6

# Embryology and development

# 20 FRCOphth best-fit MCQs

1  Which of the following structures is *not* derived from surface ectoderm?
   a. Gland of Moll
   b. Corneal epithelium
   c. Levator palpabrae superioris
   d. Lens

2  Bergmeister's papilla is a remnant of which of the following structures?
   a. Lens placode
   b. Hyaloid artery
   c. Pupillary membrane
   d. Paraxial mesoderm

3  Which of the following structures is *not* derived from the outer neuroblastic layer during development of the neurosensory retina?
   a. Amacrine cells
   b. Horizontal cells
   c. Bipolar cells
   d. Nuclei of rods and cones

4  Which of the following structures does *not* include neural crest cell-derived tissue?
   a. Ciliary epithelium
   b. Trabecular meshwork
   c. Corneal stroma
   d. Corneal endothelium

5  Which of the following congenital anomalies is *not* due to failure of closure of the optic fissure?
   a. Iris coloboma
   b. Optic nerve coloboma
   c. Lid coloboma
   d. Choroidal coloboma

6 Zonules are derived from which of the following stages of vitreous development?
  a. Primary vitreous
  b. Secondary vitreous
  c. Tertiary vitreous
  d. Quaternary vitreous

7 Which of the following vessels is derived from the ventral ophthalmic artery?
  a. Temporal long posterior ciliary artery
  b. Central retinal artery
  c. Short posterior ciliary arteries
  d. Nasal long posterior ciliary artery

8 The maxillary branch of the trigeminal nerve is derived from which pharyngeal arch?
  a. 1
  b. 2
  c. 4
  d. 6

9 The iris musculature is derived from which embryonic germ cell layer?
  a. Mesenchyme
  b. Neural crest cells
  c. Neuroectoderm
  d. Surface ectoderm

10 The optic vesicle is formed by a lateral out-pouching from which structure?
  a. Mesencephalon
  b. Diencephalon
  c. Telencephalon
  d. Rhombencephalon

11 After conception, when do the optic cups first appear?
  a. Day 23
  b. Day 25
  c. Day 27
  d. Day 33

**12** What is the length of a typical embryo at day 27 (end of week 4 post-conception)?
   **a.** 2 mm
   **b.** 5 mm
   **c.** 9 mm
   **d.** 15 mm

**13** Which of the following embryonic structures determines the final diameter of the cornea?
   **a.** Optic cup diameter
   **b.** Optic vesicle diameter
   **c.** Lens vesicle diameter
   **d.** Lens plate diameter

**14** At what stage of development are cones fully developed anatomically?
   **a.** 6 months' gestation
   **b.** Term
   **c.** 6 months
   **d.** Age 6 years

**15** Which of the following tasks would a normally developing 6-month-old be *most likely* to perform?
   **a.** Stack blocks
   **b.** Sit up
   **c.** Crawl
   **d.** Walk

**16** Which of the following methods of assessing visual acuity is most appropriate in a normally developing 3-year-old?
   **a.** LogMAR chart
   **b.** Kay's pictures
   **c.** Cardiff cards
   **d.** Fix and follow

**17** Which of the following visual acuity tests is most appropriate for detecting amblyopia?
   **a.** Crowded Kay pictures
   **b.** Cardiff cards
   **c.** Sheridan Gardiner single optotypes
   **d.** Optokinetic nystagmus

**18** In the developing foetus, what is the most common ocular complication associated with maternal rubella during the first trimester of pregnancy?
   a. Conjunctivitis
   b. Dacroadenitis
   c. Cataract
   d. Microphthalmos

**19** When does the eyeball reach its maximum size?
   a. 3 years
   b. 8 years
   c. 18 years
   d. Grows throughout life

**20** Which of the following genes inhibit apoptosis?
   a. *p53*
   b. *Bcl-2*
   c. *BAX*
   d. *Fas*

# 20 ICO true/false MCQs

21 Regarding the derivation of ocular muscles, which of the following statements are true and which are false?
  i. The superior rectus is derived from mesoderm
  ii. The medial rectus is derived from mesoderm
  iii. The pupil sphincter muscle is derived from mesoderm
  iv. The ciliary muscle is derived from mesoderm
  v. The inferior oblique muscle is derived from mesoderm

22 Regarding the development of all ocular and orbital blood vessels, which of the following statements are true and which are false?
  i. The connective tissue sheaths of blood vessels derive from neural crest cells
  ii. The muscular layer of blood vessels derives from mesoderm
  iii. The endothelial layer of blood vessels derives from mesoderm
  iv. The primitive ventral ophthalmic artery becomes the definitive ophthalmic artery
  v. Vascularisation of the nasal retina is complete before that of the temporal retina

23 Regarding the chronology of embryonic and foetal development of the eye, which of the following statements are true and which are false?
  i. Primary vitreous forms in the first month
  ii. Iris pigmentation occurs in the first trimester
  iii. The eyelids open in the second trimester
  iv. The extraocular muscles form in the third trimester
  v. The ciliary body forms in the third trimester

24 Regarding normal developmental milestones, which of the following statements are true and which are false?
  i. At birth, the baby can follow an object by head turning
  ii. At 6 weeks of age, optokinetic nystagmus can be demonstrated
  iii. By 6 months, an infant reaches well for toys
  iv. At 2 years of age, a child can identify pictures of reducing size
  v. From 5 years onwards, a child can identify a line of letters on a Snellen chart by name or matching

25 Regarding the development of the cornea, which of the following statements are true and which are false?
  i. The cornea is derived from surface ectoderm and neural crest cells
  ii. The diameter of the cornea measures 2 mm at 12 weeks' gestation
  iii. The diameter of the cornea measures 9 mm at 17 weeks' gestation
  iv. Descemet's membrane is the last of the five corneal layers to form
  v. The optic cup diameter determines the final corneal diameter

26 Regarding the development of the retina, which of the following statements are true and which are false?
  i. The neurosensory retina develops from the outer layer of the optic cup
  ii. Colour sense is developed at birth
  iii. The primitive zone divides into the inner and outer neuroblastic layers
  iv. The marginal zone contributes to the nerve fibre layer
  v. The inner neuroblastic layer gives rise to bipolar cells

27 Regarding the development of the lacrimal system, which of the following statements are true and which are false?
  i. It develops from buried buds of surface ectoderm
  ii. The lacrimal gland forms in the first trimester
  iii. Babies produce tears from birth
  iv. The lacrimal drainage system opens in the first trimester
  v. The proximal part, the punctum, is the last part of the drainage system to open

28 Regarding ocular structures derived from neural crest cells, which of the following statements are true and which are false?
  i. Corneal endothelium
  ii. Stroma of choroid
  iii. Uveal melanocytes
  iv. Corneal epithelium
  v. Retinal pigment epithelium

**29** Regarding the development of amblyopia, which of the following statements are true and which are false?

   i. Strabismic amblyopia is due to abnormal alignment of the eyes during the critical period of development

   ii. Unilateral congenital cataract can lead to stimulus deprivation amblyopia

   iii. Anisometropic amblyopia occurs when there is a significant difference in refractive error between the eyes

   iv. In amblyopia there is a demonstrable abnormality of the optic pathways

   v. Anisometropic amblyopia cannot develop with strabismic amblyopia

**30** Regarding the development of the vitreous, which of the following statements are true and which are false?

   i. Primary vitreous is composed of ectoderm and mesoderm

   ii. Cloquet's canal refers to condensation of primary vitreous around the area of the hyaloid artery

   iii. Secondary vitreous is secreted by the retina

   iv. Tertiary vitreous is secreted by the lens

   v. Persistent hyperplasia of the primary vitreous occurs when the secondary vitreous fails to be secreted and primary vitreous fibres remain

**31** Regarding development of the fovea, which of the following statements are true and which are false?

   i. The macula area starts developing in the second month of gestation

   ii. During the seventh month of gestation there is peripheral displacement of the ganglion cells and inner nuclear layer forming the fovea centralis

   iii. The foveal cones demonstrate decreased width of inner segments compared to non-foveal cones

   iv. The foveal cones demonstrate increased length of outer segments compared to non-foveal cones

   v. The macula is fully formed at birth

**32** Regarding the optic stalk, which of the following statements are true and which are false?
  i. The optic stalk is an outgrowth of mesoderm from the brain to the retina
  ii. The optic stalk lies within the choroidal fissure
  iii. The central retinal artery enters the optic stalk 5 mm posterior to the retina
  iv. In the third trimester, nerve fibres from the ganglion cells pass into the optic stalk forming the optic nerve
  v. Coloboma of the optic nerve due to incomplete closure of the choroidal fissure is typically found at the '6 o'clock' position

**33** Regarding the neural plate, which of the following statements are true and which are false?
  i. Development of the notochord induces the overlying ectoderm to differentiate into neuroectoderm that becomes identified as the neural plate
  ii. The brain and eye develop from the most posterior region of the neural plate
  iii. Neuroectodermal cells at the apex of folds of the neural plate produce a population of neural crest cells
  iv. The neural folds begin to close at the beginning of the sixth week of gestation
  v. Neural crest cells begin to migrate as the neural tube closes

**34** Regarding structures derived from surface ectoderm, which of the following statements are true and which are false?
  i. The lens is derived from surface ectoderm
  ii. The conjunctival epithelium is derived from surface ectoderm
  iii. The lacrimal gland is derived from surface ectoderm
  iv. The trabecular meshwork is derived from surface ectoderm
  v. The lacrimal drainage system is derived from surface ectoderm

35  Regarding the hyaloid artery, which of the following statements are true and which are false?

i. The hyaloid artery is a branch of the primitive dorsal ophthalmic artery

ii. The hyaloid artery runs through the optic stalk

iii. The tunica vasculosa lentis forms an envelope around the developing lens

iv. The hyaloid artery regresses to eventually become the central retinal artery

v. The central retinal artery supplies the inner layers of the retina up to and including the outer nuclear layer of the retina

36  Regarding the lens, which of the following statements are true and which are false?

i. The lens placode is a thickening of surface ectoderm overlying the optic vesicle

ii. The lens placode is first seen at day 10 of gestation

iii. The lens vesicle separates from the surface epithelium at approximately day 33 of gestation

iv. The first suture marking the foetal nucleus is shaped like a Y posteriorly

v. The hyaloid artery supplies blood to the lens at birth

37  True or false, the *PAX6* homeobox gene is implicated in the following developmental conditions:

i. Aniridia

ii. Peters' anomaly

iii. Congenital cataract

iv. Optic nerve hypoplasia

v. Foveal hypoplasia

38  True or false, the following structures are derived from neuroectoderm:

i. Neurosensory retina

ii. Optic nerve

iii. Retinal pigment epithelium

iv. Connective tissue of iris

v. Ciliary ganglion

**39** Regarding myelination of the optic nerve, which of the following statements are true and which are false?

    **i.** Myelination begins during the seventh month of gestation

    **ii.** Myelination of the optic nerve is complete by birth

    **iii.** The retinal nerve fibre layer is myelinated

    **iv.** Myelination allows more rapid nerve conduction

    **v.** Myelination progresses posteriorly from the lamina cribosa

**40** Regarding the development of the orbit, which of the following statements are true and which are false?

    **i.** The eyeball develops entirely within the confines of the orbit

    **ii.** The orbital bones develop from mesenchyme that encircles the optic vesicle

    **iii.** The medial wall develops from the maxillary process

    **iv.** The optic axis is 105 degrees at birth

    **v.** The bones of the orbit form in membrane except those belonging to the base of the skull, which develop in cartilage

# 7
# Optics

7

Optics

# 30 FRCOphth best-fit MCQs

1  Wavelength is best defined as:
   a. One complete oscillation
   b. The maximum displacement of an imaginary particle on the wave from the baseline
   c. The distance between two symmetrical parts of the wave motion
   d. Any portion of a cycle

2  Destructive interference is seen in:
   a. Corneal epithelium
   b. Refraction
   c. Antireflective lens coatings
   d. Photochromic lenses

3  Which of the following is *not* a test of stereoacuity?
   a. Titmus
   b. Frisby
   c. Pelli-Robson
   d. TNO

4  Which of the following definitions best describes radiant flux?
   a. The amount of light emitted from a source
   b. The intensity of light emitted from a source
   c. The amount of light falling on a surface
   d. The amount of light reflected from a surface

5  The unit of illuminance is:
   a. Lumen
   b. Lux (lumen per square metre)
   c. Candelas (lumen per steradian)
   d. Watts per steradian

6  The image of an object formed by reflection at a plane surface is *not*:
   a. Erect
   b. Virtual
   c. Enlarged
   d. Laterally inverted

**7** The catoptric image formed from which of the following is inverted?
a. Anterior corneal surface
b. Posterior corneal surface
c. Anterior lens surface
d. Posterior lens surface

**8** Which of the following changes when a ray of light passes into a denser medium?
a. Velocity and frequency
b. Velocity and plane
c. Frequency and plane
d. Velocity only

**9** Total internal reflection occurs if the incident ray strikes the interface of media at:
a. An angle less than the critical angle
b. The critical angle
c. An angle greater than the critical angle
d. 90 degrees

**10** An object located between the centre of curvature and principal focus of a concave mirror is:
a. Diminished
b. Virtual
c. Erect
d. Real

**11** Which of the following does *not* determine the angle of deviation of a ray of light when refracted by a prism?
a. Refractive index of the material of which the prism is made
b. Wavelength of light of the incident ray
c. Refracting angle of the prism
d. Angle of incidence of the ray

**12** Which of the following is true regarding the image formed by a prism?
a. It is virtual and displaced towards the apex
b. It is real and displaced towards the apex
c. It is virtual and displaced towards the base
d. It is real and displaced towards the base

**13** A glass prism (refractive index 1.5) of 20 prism dioptres deviates an incident ray of light through:
   **a.** 5 degrees
   **b.** 10 degrees
   **c.** 20 degrees
   **d.** 40 degrees

**14** For a convex lens, placing an object inside the first principal focus $(F_1)$ results in an image that is:
   **a.** Enlarged, inverted and real
   **b.** Enlarged, erect and real
   **c.** Enlarged, inverted and virtual
   **d.** Enlarged, erect and virtual

**15** If a 10-dioptre concave lens is decentred by 2 cm temporally, this will result in a:
   **a.** 5 prism dioptre base-in prism
   **b.** 5 prism dioptre base-out prism
   **c.** 20 prism dioptre base-in prism
   **d.** 20 prism dioptre base-out prism

**16** The spherical equivalent of a lens with power +3.00 DS/–2.00 DC is:
   **a.** +1.00 DS
   **b.** +2.00 DS
   **c.** –0.50 DS
   **d.** –1.00 DS

**17** Transpose the –4.00 DS/–3.00 DC × 45 into positive cylinder notation:
   **a.** –5.50 DS/+3.00 DC × 45
   **b.** –5.50 DS/+3.00 DC × 135
   **c.** –7.00 DS/+300 DC × 135
   **d.** –7.00 DS/+3.00 DC × 45

**18** Transpose +2.00 DS/–1.00 DC × 180 to the base curve –2 D:

   **a.** $$\frac{+4.00 \text{ DS}}{-2.00 \text{ DC} \times 90/-3.00 \text{ DC} \times 180}$$

   **b.** $$\frac{+4.00 \text{ DS}}{-3.00 \text{ DC} \times 90/-3.00 \text{ DC} \times 180}$$

   **c.** $$\frac{+4.00 \text{ DS}}{-2.00 \text{ DC} \times 90/+1.00 \text{ DC} \times 180}$$

   **d.** $$\frac{+4.00 \text{ DS}}{-2.00 \text{ DC} \times 90/-1.00 \text{ DC} \times 180}$$

**19** Which of the following is *not* a means for reducing spherical aberration?
  **a.** Use of stops
  **b.** Aplanatic surfaces
  **c.** Pantoscopic tilt
  **d.** Use of a doublet

**20** Which of the following is *not* a problem with spectacle correction of aphakia?
  **a.** Image magnification
  **b.** Ring scotoma
  **c.** Pin-cushion distortion
  **d.** Barrel distortion

**21** Based on Gullstrand's reduced eye, which of the following points is 7.08 mm behind the anterior corneal surface?
  **a.** Nodal point
  **b.** Principal point
  **c.** First focal point
  **d.** Second focal point

**22** The crystalline lens has an effective power in situ of:
  **a.** 15 dioptres
  **b.** 23 dioptres
  **c.** 37 dioptres
  **d.** 43 dioptres

**23** Which of the following definitions is *not* correct?
  **a.** The near point is the point at which an object can be clearly seen when maximum accommodation is used
  **b.** The range of accommodation is the distance between the far point and near point
  **c.** The amplitude of accommodation is the dioptric power difference between the eye at rest and when fully accommodated
  **d.** The dioptric power of the accommodated eye is called its static refraction

**24** A high AC/A ratio may be associated with:
  **a.** Divergence excess esotropia
  **b.** Convergence excess esotropia
  **c.** Convergence weakness
  **d.** Convergence excess exotropia

**25** Keratoconus can cause:
   a. Axial myopia
   b. Refractive myopia
   c. Axial hypermetropia
   d. Refractive hypermetropia

**26** If rays of light from all meridians come into focus behind the retina, this is called:
   a. Simple myopic astigmatism
   b. Compound myopic astigmatism
   c. Simple hypermetropic astigmatism
   d. Compound hypermetropic astigmatism

**27** In a hypermetropic eye, by moving a convex lens away from the eye:
   a. The effectivity of the lens is decreased
   b. The effectivity of the lens is increased
   c. The effectivity of the lens is unchanged
   d. None of the above

**28** A hypermetrope whose glasses contain +5.00 DS lenses wants to wear contact lenses. What is the dioptric power of the contact lens that he would require? (Back vertex distance = 15 mm.)
   a. 4.5 dioptres
   b. 5.0 dioptres
   c. 5.4 dioptres
   d. 5.8 dioptres

**29** An eye has axial length 23.0 mm, with average keratometry readings of 42 dioptres. Using the SRK formula (A constant 118.9), aiming for emmetropia, the calculated power of an intraocular lens implant would be:
   a. 23.6 dioptres
   b. 25.3 dioptres
   c. 26.3 dioptres
   d. 26.6 dioptres

**30** Which of the following does *not* decrease the tolerability of progressive addition lenses:
   a. Large cylinder
   b. High reading addition
   c. Wide progression corridor
   d. Smaller distance and near portions

# 30 ICO true/false MCQs

**31** Which of the following may be corrected using corneal contact lenses?
   **i.** Regular astigmatism of 1.50 dioptres
   **ii.** Aphakia
   **iii.** Presbyopia
   **iv.** 2 dioptre exotropia
   **v.** 1 dioptre hypertropia

**32** Which of the following combinations of lenses can be used to make a Galilean telescope?
   **i.** +2.5 dioptre objective and −10 dioptre eyepiece lens separated by 30 cm
   **ii.** −2.5 dioptre objective and +10 dioptre eyepiece lens separated by 20 cm
   **iii.** +4 dioptre objective and −20 dioptre eyepiece lens separated by 30 cm
   **iv.** −4 dioptre objective and −20 dioptre eyepiece lens separated by 30 cm
   **v.** +4 dioptre objective and −20 dioptre eyepiece lens separated by 20 cm

**33** Which of the following factors limit magnifiers as low visual aids for distance vision?
   **i.** Need to be held close to the eye
   **ii.** Reduced field of view
   **iii.** Increased depth of focus
   **iv.** Unsteadiness of hand
   **v.** Virtual image

**34** Which of the following types of refractive surgery can be used effectively for correction of high myopia (−6 dioptres)?
   **i.** Photorefractive keratotomy
   **ii.** Radial keratotomy
   **iii.** Thermokeratoplasty
   **iv.** Epikeratophakia
   **v.** Laser intrastromal keratomileusis

**35** Which of the following statements regarding vitreoretinal surgery are true and which are false?

   **i.** Silicone oil fill in a phakic eye causes myopic shift

   **ii.** Silicone oil fill in an aphakic eye causes myopic shift

   **iii.** Gas fill in a phakic eye causes a myopic shift

   **iv.** Gas fill in an aphakic eye causes a myopic shift

   **v.** Use of scleral buckles causes myopic shift

**36** Regarding colour vision, which of the following statements are true and which are false?

   **i.** Light of wavelength 300–780 nm is transmitted through the ocular media to the retina

   **ii.** UVA light is absorbed by the lens

   **iii.** The blue opsin gene is on chromosome 7

   **iv.** Protanopia describes an absence of green cone function

   **v.** Deuteranomaly describes a shift in blue cone sensitivity

**37** Regarding properties of light, which of the following statements are true and which are false?

   **i.** Fluorescence is a property where a molecule can spontaneously emit light of a shorter wavelength when stimulated by light of a longer wavelength

   **ii.** Fluorescein emits light of wavelength 520–530 nm when stimulated

   **iii.** A polarised beam of light is one in which the individual wave motions lie perpendicular to each other

   **iv.** Birefringent substances transmit light waves lying parallel to their structure but redirect light waves that are perpendicular

   **v.** Dichroic substances reflect light waves not aligned with their structure

**38** Regarding the image formed when light is reflected by a convex mirror, which of the following statements are true and which are false?

   **i.** The image is virtual

   **ii.** The image is smaller than the object

   **iii.** The image is laterally inverted

   **iv.** The image is inverted if the object is located outside the centre of curvature

   **v.** The image is inverted if the object is located between the centre of curvature and principal focus

**39** Regarding refraction of light at a curved surface:
  i. Snell's law is obeyed
  ii. If the refractive index of the medium the light enters into is higher than the original medium, light is converged to a focus
  iii. If the refractive index of the medium the light enters into is lower than the original medium, light is converged to a focus
  iv. The surface refracting power of a curved surface is proportional to its radius of curvature
  v. Surface power is given a negative sign for diverging surfaces and a positive sign for converging surfaces

**40** Regarding refraction by prisms, which of the following statements are true and which are false?
  i. In the Prentice position, the angle of incidence is equal to the angle of emergence
  ii. The Prentice position power is normally specified for glass prisms such as in trial lenses
  iii. The refractive index of glass is 1.5
  iv. The refractive power of prisms stacked on top of one another is the same as the sum of the refractive powers of the individual prisms
  v. A prism of power-two prism dioptres deviates light through 2 degrees

**41** Regarding prisms in clinical use:
  i. Fresnel prisms are permanent prisms incorporated into spectacle lenses
  ii. When prescribing prisms, they are usually only incorporated into one of the spectacle lenses
  iii. Base-out prisms are used to treat convergence insufficiency
  iv. The apex of the prisms is placed in the direction of deviation of the eye
  v. Prisms may be used to assess cases of fictitious blindness

**42** Which of the following properties are true regarding the image formed by a thin concave lens?
  i. It is virtual
  ii. It is erect
  iii. It is smaller than the object
  iv. It is positioned between the second principal focus and the lens
  v. It is laterally inverted

**43** Regarding the prismatic power that results following decentration of a spherical lens:

    i. Prism power is directly proportional to decentration

    ii. Prism power is inversely proportional to power of the spherical lens

    iii. A concave lens decentred nasally results in a base-in prism

    iv. A convex lens decentred superiorly results in a base-up prism

    v. A convex lens decentred temporally results in a base-out prism

**44** Regarding the Maddox rod, which of the following statements are true and which are false?

    i. It is composed of several concave cylindrical lenses

    ii. When viewed through a Maddox rod, a linear object is seen as a point image

    iii. The object must be placed at least 6 metres away from the patient

    iv. Incident light that is parallel to the cylinders in the Maddox rod are brought to focus in front of the eye

    v. Incident light that is perpendicular to the cylinders in the Maddox rod are brought to focus on the retina

**45** Regarding toric lenses, which of the following statements are true and which are false?

    i. The cylindrical surface is curved in both horizontal and vertical meridians

    ii. The principal meridian of maximum curvature is called the base curve

    iii. Each meridian of curvature forms a separate line focus

    iv. −2.00 DS/+1.00 DC has a spherical equivalent of −1.00 DS

    v. +3.00 DS/+2.00 DC has a spherical equivalent of +4.00 DS

**46** Regarding identification of spectacle lens type, which of the following statements are true and which are false?

    i. When a convex lens is placed over a cross and moved from side to side, the cross that is seen moves with the direction of movement

    ii. When a concave lens is placed over a cross and moved from side to side, the cross that is seen moves with the direction of movement

    iii. When a toric lens is placed over a cross and moved from side to side, the cross that is seen is distorted

    iv. A prismatic lens can be centred over both arms of the cross

    v. A Geneva lens measure is calibrated for plastic lenses

**47** Regarding the duochrome test, which of the following statements are true and which are false?

i. The test is able to detect an alteration in refraction of 1 dioptre or less

ii. A myope sees the letters on the red background more clearly

iii. A hypermetrope sees the letters on the green background more clearly

iv. At the end of subjective refraction, a myope should be left seeing the letters on the green background slightly better

v. The test cannot be used in colour-blind patients

**48** Regarding oblique astigmatism, which of the following statements are true and which are false?

i. It occurs when the incident light is not parallel to the principal axis of the lens

ii. It may be reduced by pantoscopic tilt of spectacle lenses

iii. It is less problematic in biconvex or biconcave lenses

iv. It is reduced in the eye by the aplanatic nature of the cornea

v. It is reduced in the eye by the curved nature of the retina

**49** Regarding hypermetropia, which of the following statements are true and which are false?

i. Refractive hypermetropia may be caused by aphakia

ii. Manifest hypermetropia occurs when the eye is too short for its refractive power

iii. Latent hypermetropia is the residual hypermetropia that is involuntarily corrected for by ciliary tone and accommodation

iv. Facultative hypermetropia is that which can be overcome by accommodation

v. Absolute hypermetropia is the strongest convex lens correction that can be accepted for clear distance vision

**50** If an emmetropic person has 3 dioptres remaining amplitude of accommodation, the presbyopic correction required is:

i. 1.0 dioptre to read clearly at 50 cm

ii. 2.0 dioptres to read clearly at 25 cm

iii. 3.0 dioptres to read clearly at 20 cm

iv. 3.5 dioptres to read clearly at 15 cm

v. 5.0 dioptres to read clearly at 10 cm

51 Regarding the Stiles-Crawford effect, which of the following statements are true and which are false?
   i. It reduces chromatic aberration in the eye
   ii. It reduces spherical aberration in the eye
   iii. It affects photopic vision more than scotopic vision
   iv. It involves the directional sensitivity of rods
   v. The troland measure of illumination includes correction for the Stiles-Crawford effect

52 Regarding spectacle correction of aphakia:
   i. It has a magnification effect of 1.33
   ii. Objects appear to be further away than they really are
   iii. This may result in enhanced performance in Snellen visual acuity testing
   iv. The heavy lenses may slip down the patient's nose, decreasing their effectivity
   v. Pin-cushion distortion may be seen

53 To leave them emmetropic, what power of intraocular lens (A constant 118.0) will be required for a patient with axial length 22.1 mm and average keratometry readings of 43 dioptres (using the SRK formula)?
   i. 22.5 dioptres
   ii. 23.0 dioptres
   iii. 23.5 dioptres
   iv. 24.0 dioptres
   v. 24.5 dioptres

54 Which of the following will reduce 'with the rule' astigmatism in a patient undergoing cataract surgery?
   i. A superior corneal incision
   ii. A temporal corneal incision
   iii. A toric intraocular lens with positive power in the 90-degree meridian
   iv. Limbal relaxing incisions centred on the 90-degree meridian
   v. An arcuate keratotomy centred on the 180-degree meridian

55 Which of the following tests can be used to test colour vision?
   i. Farnsworth-Munsell test
   ii. D-15 test
   iii. VISITECH chart
   iv. Vernier acuity
   v. Ishihara test

**56** Regarding an 8-dioptre biconvex spherical lens, which of the following statements are true and which are false?

   **i.** It is a converging lens
   **ii.** It has positive vergence power
   **iii.** It has a focal length of 20 cm
   **iv.** It can be used in a magnifying loupe
   **v.** If the lens is decentred by 2 cm, it has a prismatic power of 16 dioptres

**57** Regarding retinoscopy reflexes:

   **i.** If a 'with movement' is seen, further concave lenses must be added
   **ii.** If an 'against movement' is seen, further convex lenses must be added
   **iii.** If the reflex moves obliquely off axis, astigmatism has not been neutralised
   **iv.** A swirling reflex can be seen near the endpoint of retinoscopy
   **v.** A scissor reflex is a sign of keratoconus

**58** If a Maddox rod is placed in front of the right eye, what condition does the patient have if the image seen of a point source of light is:

   **i.** Orthophoria
   **ii.** Exophoria
   **iii.** Esophoria
   **iv.** Right hyperphoria
   **v.** Right hypophoria

**59** If an object is placed outside the first principal focus, the image formed by a thin convex lens is:

   **i.** Real
   **ii.** Virtual
   **iii.** Inverted
   **iv.** Erect
   **v.** Inside the second principal focus

**60** Unilateral spectacle correction of aphakia, in an adult, may leave the patient with:

   **i.** Amblyopia
   **ii.** Anisometropia
   **iii.** Aniseikonia
   **iv.** Diplopia
   **v.** Astigmatism

# 8
# Therapeutics

# 20 FRCOphth best-fit MCQs

1 Which of the following factors increases ocular absorption of topical medication?
   a. Use of an ointment instead of drops
   b. Hydrophilic medications
   c. Reflex tearing
   d. Administration of multiple drops of medication

2 Patients with very pigmented irides dilate poorly with atropine due to:
   a. First-order kinetics
   b. Zero-order kinetics
   c. Active transport
   d. Tissue binding

3 Which of the following antibiotics has good ocular penetration when given orally:
   a. Ciprofloxacin
   b. Co-amoxiclav
   c. Cephalexin
   d. Cephradine

4 Which one of the following effects is caused by stimulation of adrenergic receptors in the eye?
   a. Pupil constriction
   b. Pupil dilation
   c. Conjunctival blood vessel dilation
   d. Ptosis

5 Which of the following is a side effect of beta-2 receptor blockade?
   a. Asthma attacks
   b. Hypotension
   c. Bradycardia
   d. Increased intraocular pressure

6 Apraclonidine:
   a. Is a relatively selective alpha-1 agonist
   b. Crosses the blood-brain barrier
   c. Is not used for long-term treatment
   d. May cause increased salivation

7 Which of the following statements is true regarding pilocarpine?
   a. Will reverse a mydriasis caused by administration of phenylephrine
   b. Is a direct nicotinic acetylcholine receptor agonist
   c. May cause accommodative spasm
   d. Reduces risk of retinal tears

8 Which of the following mydriatics does *not* inhibit accommodation?
   a. Atropine
   b. Tropicamide
   c. Cyclopentolate
   d. Phenylephrine

9 Acetazolamide:
   a. Can be given to patients with allergy to sulphasalazine
   b. Acts on the non-pigmented ciliary epithelium to inhibit aqueous production
   c. May cause a metabolic alkalosis
   d. Can cause a transient hypermetropia

10 Mannitol:
   a. Acts by reducing the osmotic pressure of plasma relative to aqueous and vitreous
   b. Cannot be used in diabetics
   c. May cause pulmonary oedema
   d. Can be given orally or intravenously

11 Latanoprost:
   a. Acts via prostaglandin receptors
   b. Acts by reducing aqueous production
   c. Increases melanogenesis
   d. Should be used with caution in patients with asthma

12 Histamine receptor blockade may cause:
   a. Bronchospasm
   b. Vasodilation
   c. Reduced production of gastric acid
   d. Positive chronotropic effect on the heart

13 Glucocorticoids act via:
   a. G-protein coupled receptors
   b. Cytosolic receptors
   c. Ligand-gated ion channels
   d. Receptors with protein-tyrosine-kinase activity

14 The majority of non-steroidal anti-inflammatory medications work by:
   a. Inhibiting prostaglandin synthesis
   b. Inhibiting leukotriene synthesis
   c. Inhibiting histamine production
   d. Inhibiting free radical scavenging mechanisms

15 5-Fluorouracil:
   a. Is a purine analogue
   b. Is a pyrimidine analogue
   c. Is an alkylating agent
   d. Targets non-dividing cells

16 Cyclosporin A:
   a. Acts via B-cell inhibition
   b. May be nephrotoxic
   c. Is metabolised by the kidney
   d. May cause gum hypoplasia

17 Lignocaine:
   a. Has a longer-lasting action than Marcaine
   b. Is weakly acidic
   c. Prevents influx of sodium ions across axonal membranes
   d. Is mainly metabolised by the kidney

18 Suxamethonium:
   a. Is a non-depolarising blocker of the neuromuscular junction
   b. Is not reversed by administering anticholinesterase inhibitors
   c. May cause hypokalaemia
   d. May cause ocular hypotony

**19** Regarding botulinum toxin:
   **a.** It potentiates release of acetylcholine from motor nerve terminals
   **b.** There are eight known serotypes
   **c.** Serotype C is used in clinical practice
   **d.** Administration may induce a permanent ptosis

**20** Use of which of the following medications is associated with development of cataract?
   **a.** Ethambutol
   **b.** Amiodarone
   **c.** Vigabatrin
   **d.** Glucocorticoids

# 20 ICO true/false MCQs

**21** Which of the following statements regarding drug antagonism are true and which are false?
  **i.** In non-competitive antagonism both drugs bind to the same receptor
  **ii.** Non-competitive antagonism may be reversible or irreversible
  **iii.** In irreversible competitive antagonism, the antagonist dissociates very slowly or not at all from drug receptors
  **iv.** In pharmacokinetic antagonism, one drug affects the absorption, metabolism or excretion of another
  **v.** In physiological antagonism, two drugs with opposing actions in the body cancel each other out

**22** Regarding G-protein coupled receptors:
  **i.** G-proteins are membrane bound
  **ii.** Binding of an agonist to a receptor activates a single G-protein molecule
  **iii.** The G-protein beta subunit catalyses the conversion of GTP to GDP
  **iv.** Nicotinic acetylcholine receptors are an example
  **v.** Beta-adrenoreceptors are an example

**23** Regarding local anaesthesia for cataract surgery, which of the following statements are true and which are false?
  **i.** Globe and conjunctival anaesthesia are achieved by blockade of the ophthalmic and mandibular branches of the trigeminal nerve
  **ii.** All methods of delivery of anaesthesia also cause akinesia
  **iii.** Sub-Tenon's anaesthesia is contraindicated in high myopia
  **iv.** High doses of topical anaesthesia may cause corneal erosion
  **v.** Peribulbar block may cause proptosis

**24** Regarding azathioprine, which of the following statements are true and which are false?
  **i.** It acts via inhibiting pyrimidine synthesis
  **ii.** It may be used in the treatment of thyroid eye disease
  **iii.** Full blood count must be regularly monitored during its use
  **iv.** Urea and electrolytes must be regularly monitored during its use
  **v.** Serum levels of TPMT enzyme should be checked prior to commencing treatment

**25** Regarding brimonidine, which of the following statements are true and which are false?
  **i.** It is a beta-2 agonist
  **ii.** It is more effective than latanoprost
  **iii.** It causes mydriasis
  **iv.** It may cause dry mouth
  **v.** It may cause blepharoconjunctivitis

**26** In which of the following drugs is tachyphylaxis a significant concern?
  **i.** Latanoprost
  **ii.** Apraclonidine
  **iii.** Dorzolamide
  **iv.** Brimonidine
  **v.** Timolol

**27** Regarding dorzolamide, which of the following statements are true and which are false?
  **i.** It is a topical carbonic anhydrase agonist
  **ii.** It acts by increasing uveoscleral outflow
  **iii.** It is contraindicated in patients with sulphonamide allergy
  **iv.** Side effects include a bitter taste
  **v.** It may cause periorbital contact dermatitis

**28** Which of the following side effects are associated with oral antihistamines?
  **i.** Miosis
  **ii.** Epiphora
  **iii.** Urinary retention
  **iv.** Palpitations
  **v.** Drowsiness

**29** Regarding benzalkonium chloride, which of the following statements are true and which are false?

   **i.** It is a commonly used preservative in eye drops

   **ii.** It is bacteriostatic

   **iii.** It is most effective at an acidic pH

   **iv.** It is largely non-toxic to the corneal epithelium

   **v.** It is activated in the presence of calcium

**30** Regarding ocular side effects of systemic drugs, which of the following statements are true and which are false?

   **i.** Amiodarone may cause vortex keratopathy

   **ii.** Tamoxifen may cause maculopathy

   **iii.** Hydroxychloroquine is more likely to cause retinal toxicity than chloroquine

   **iv.** Gentamicin injected intravitreally may cause retinal ischaemia

   **v.** Ethambutol may cause optic neuropathy

**31** Which of the following statements are true and which are false regarding ocular topical corticosteroids?

   **i.** They most commonly are associated with anterior cortical cataract

   **ii.** They may act via steroid receptors located on the trabecular meshwork to raise intraocular pressure

   **ii.** Raised intraocular pressure is more likely if the patient is hypermetropic

   **iii.** They may cause central serous retinopathy

   **v.** They may cause scleral thinning

**32** Regarding ligand-gated ion channels, which of the following statements are true and which are false?

   **i.** They are transmembrane proteins

   **ii.** They are mainly involved in events controlling cell growth and differentiation

   **iii.** Channel opening is rapid

   **iv.** GABA A channels are an example

   **v.** Muscarinic acetylcholine receptors are an example

**33** Regarding drug metabolism, which of the following statements are true and which are false?

    i. Phase I reactions involve oxidation, reduction or hydrolysis

    ii. Phase II reactions involve conjugation

    iii. Phase II reactions often involve the P450 enzyme system in the liver

    iv. Drugs that induce liver enzymes lead to reduced drug metabolism

    v. First-pass metabolism usually involves renal excretion

**34** Which of the following may be caused by use of non-steroidal anti-inflammatory drugs?

    i. Gastric ulceration

    ii. Acute renal failure

    iii. Hepatitis

    iv. Increased risk of stroke

    v. Bone marrow suppression

**35** Genetic polymorphisms can influence metabolism of which of the following drugs?

    i. Azathioprine

    ii. Isoniazid

    iii. Dapsone

    iv. Erythromycin

    v. Ciprofloxacin

**36** Which of the following combinations of intravitreal antibiotics are recommended for the treatment of endophthalmitis?

    i. Amikacin and gentamicin

    ii. Vancomycin and amikacin

    iii. Vancomycin and ceftazidime

    iv. Ceftazidime and gentamicin

    iv. Ceftazidime and amikacin

**37** Which of the following drugs show zero-order (or saturation) kinetics?

    i. Aspirin

    ii. Phenytoin

    iii. Amiodarone

    iv. Propranolol

    v. Ciprofloxacin

**38** Regarding methotrexate, which of the following statements are true and which are false?
  i. It is a folate agonist
  ii. It is excreted by the liver
  iii. It may cause bone marrow depression
  iv. It may cause abnormal liver function tests
  v. It may be used in the treatment of scleritis

**39** Regarding opiates, which of the following statements and which are false?
  i. They act via α- and β-receptors
  ii. Pupil constriction is mediated by stimulation of iris opioid receptors
  iii. They may cause respiratory depression
  iv. They may cause diarrhoea
  v. They may cause cough suppression

**40** Which of the following side effects may be caused by acetazolamide?
  i. Paraesthesiae
  ii. Metallic taste
  iii. Metabolic alkalosis
  iv. Thrombocytosis
  v. Aplastic anaemia

# 9
# Lasers and instruments

# 25 FRCOphth best-fit MCQs

1 Which of the following wavelengths is most likely *not* to penetrate the eye?
   a. 380 μm
   b. 500 μm
   c. 650 μm
   d. 1200 μm

2 The fundus camera in fluorescein angiography uses the following filters:
   a. Blue excitation and green barrier filter
   b. Green excitation and blue barrier filter
   c. Yellow excitation and blue barrier filter
   d. Blue excitation and yellow barrier filter

3 The following laser energy is well absorbed by melanin and haemoglobin:
   a. Argon blue-green
   b. Diode laser
   c. Nd-YAG
   d. Holmium

4 Rose Bengal is best seen using the following filter on slit-lamp examination:
   a. Blue cobalt
   b. Red free
   c. Neutral density
   d. Unfiltered

5 The magnification achieved by the direct ophthalmoscope is typically:
   a. 4 x
   b. 15 x
   c. 50 x
   d. 8 x

6 Therapeutic lasers used in ophthalmology are classified as:
   a. Class 1
   b. Class 0
   c. Class 3b or 4
   d. Class 2 or 3a

7  Laser pumping:
   a. Allows the release of atoms
   b. Congregates atoms
   c. Elevates an atom to a higher energy state
   d. Involves spontaneous decay

8  Using an indirect ophthalmoscope, the image viewed by the observer will be:
   a. Virtual, vertically and laterally inverted
   b. Real, and vertically inverted
   c. Real, vertically and laterally inverted
   d. Virtual and laterally inverted

9  The power of a laser is most likely to be increased by:
   a. Decreasing the shutter speed
   b. Being in continuous waveform
   c. Being in fundamental mode
   d. Q-switching

10 The following type of laser is best suited to measuring the retinal nerve fibre layer thickness:
   a. Scanning laser polarimetry
   b. Confocal scanning laser tomography
   c. Laser interferometry
   d. Confocal microscopy

11 An emmetropic observer elects to view the retina of a patient using the direct ophthalmoscope. The patient is 55 years of age, has uncorrected vision of 6/36 and tells the observer he has an astigmatism of 1.25D. To obtain a clear view of the fundus, he dials –6.0D on the ophthalmoscope. What is the most likely scenario?
   a. The patient is –6.0D myopic
   b. The observer is accommodating to view the retina
   c. The patient is +6.0D hypermetropic
   d. The observer is not emmetropic

12 Photodynamic therapy with verteporfin is best used for treatment in:
   a. Occult choroidal neovascular membrane
   b. Classic subfoveal age-related macular degeneration
   c. Disciform age-related macular degeneration
   d. Rubeosis iridis

**13** A corneal pachymeter can be best described by using:
   **a.** Purkinje-Sanson images II and III
   **b.** Purkinje-Sanson images I and II
   **c.** Purkinje-Sanson images III and IV
   **d.** Purkinje-Sanson images I and IV

**14** Using a compound microscope the image is:
   **a.** Real, upright and magnified
   **b.** Real, upright and minified
   **c.** Real, inverted and magnified
   **d.** Real, inverted and minified

**15** Regarding the Javal-Schiotz keratometer:
   **a.** It has a fixed image size and is typically a two-position instrument
   **b.** It has a variable image size
   **c.** It has a variable image size and is typically a two-position instrument
   **d.** It has a fixed image size and is typically a one-position instrument

**16** The following is *not* an example of a contact lens:
   **a.** Koeppe lens
   **b.** Rodenstock lens
   **c.** Hruby lens
   **d.** Mainster lens

**17** Using the Goldmann applanation tonometer, the intraocular pressure reading is likely to be artificially elevated by:
   **a.** Pseudophakia
   **b.** Absent corneal astigmatism
   **c.** Thin cornea
   **d.** Thick cornea

**18** In a Humphrey visual field analysis, the following condition may result in decreased mean deviation:
   **a.** Keratoconus
   **b.** Cataract
   **c.** Poor tear film
   **d.** Gorlin-Goltz syndrome

**19** Which light is used in a focimeter and why?
  a. Blue light to limit spherical aberration
  b. Green light to limit spherical aberration
  c. Blue light to limit chromatic aberration
  d. Green light to limit chromatic aberration

**20** The Geneva Lens Measure measures the surface power of the lens by:
  a. Measuring the surface curvature
  b. Measuring the diameter
  c. Measuring the thickness of the lens
  d. Measuring the total volume of the lens

**21** The following is an example of a kinetic perimeter:
  a. Humphrey
  b. Simmons
  c. Goldmann
  d. Frequency doubling

**22** A disadvantage of the Tono-Pen is that:
  a. It can only be used once
  b. It requires extensive training to use
  c. It is less accurate than the Goldmann tonometer
  d. It requires a mains electrical connection

**23** Using a streak retinoscope with the shaft down and a working distance of 0.5 m, in a high hypermetrope:
  a. The luminous reflex will move in the same direction as the retinoscopy movement
  b. The luminous reflex will move in the opposite direction to the retinoscopy movement
  c. Scissoring reflex will be seen
  d. Oil-droplet reflex will be seen

**24** Using the indirect ophthalmoscope, the most important determinants of the field of view are:
  a. The subject's pupil size and distance between the subject and the condensing lens
  b. The observer's pupil size and the distance between the observer and the condensing lens
  c. The subject's pupil size and the distance between the observer and the condensing lens
  d. The diameter of the condensing lens and the observer's pupil size

**25** Optical coherence tomography typically uses:
   **a.** Ultraviolet B
   **b.** Green light
   **c.** Infrared light
   **d.** Microwaves

# 25 ICO true/false MCQs

**26** Regarding the indirect ophthalmoscope, which of the following statements are true and which are false?

   i. A stereoscopic view is possible unlike with the direct ophthalmoscope

   ii. The eyepieces usually contain +2D lenses

   iii. The image is not inverted

   iv. The field of view is independent of the refractive error of the patient

   v. A higher-power condensing lens produces a smaller field of view

**27** Regarding the direct ophthalmoscope, which of the following statements are true and which are false?

   i. The magnification is independent of the refractive error of the patient

   ii. A red filter is useful for examining the retinal vasculature

   iii. It can correct for astigmatism

   iv. Reducing the spot size is useful for small pupils

   v. An erect virtual image of the retina is seen

**28** Regarding keratometry, which of the following statements are true and which are false?

   i. It provides measurements for curvature of the peripheral cornea only

   ii. It provides measurements for the curvature of the lens

   iii. Two readings are usually taken with the Javal-Schiotz keratometer

   iv. Four readings are usually taken with the Helmholtz keratometer

   v. Eyes with regular astigmatism will not allow readings 90 degrees to each other

**29** Regarding the focimeter, which of the following statements are true and which are false?

   i. It measures the crystalline lens power

   ii. It measures spectacle lens power

   iii. The power of the cylindrical correction is equivalent to the difference between the first and second power readings

   iv. It cannot measure bifocal lenses

   v. If the image cannot be centred, the patient may have diplopia

**30** Regarding indocyanine green (ICG) angiography, which of the following statements are true and which are false?

   i. Is useful in studying choroidal disease

   ii. 48% of ICG molecules bind to proteins in the blood

   iii. The excitation peak for ICG is 445 nm

   iv. ICG should not be given to patients allergic to iodine

   v. Pruritis is an extremely rare side effect

**31** Which of the following ophthalmic instruments can examine the anterior chamber angle?

   i. The Hruby lens

   ii. The 28D lens

   iii. The Koeppe lens

   iv. The Goldmann three-mirror lens

   v. The Panfundscope lens

**32** Which of the following instruments may be used to check intraocular pressure?

   i. The Javal-Schiotz tonometer

   ii. The Perkins tonometer

   iii. The Goldmann tonometer

   iv. The Tono-Pen

   v. The air-puff tonometer

**33** The Oculus Pentacam instrument is:

   i. Useful for assessment of patients with keratoconus

   ii. Useful for patients undergoing refractive surgery

   iii. Useful for patients with basal cell carcinoma

   iv. Useful for patients with glaucoma

   v. Useful for patients with advanced macular degeneration

**34** Regarding Goldmann perimetry, which of the following statements are true and which are false?

   i. It is inaccurate in children

   ii. It is useful for the detection of neurological conditions

   iii. The patient is not required to maintain fixation

   iv. Dimmer lights are used to assess sensitivity thresholds

   v. The blind spot is not mapped

**35** Regarding colour vision, which of the following statements are true and which are false?
  i. Using Ishihara colour-vision testing, only those with normal colour vision will see plates 10 and 17
  ii. Ishihara colour-vision testing cannot screen congenital red/green defects
  iii. Innumerate patients cannot be tested with Ishihara colour-vision testing
  iv. The Farnsworth-Munsell 100-hue test can detect mild colour-vision abnormalities and contains 100 movable tiles
  v. The Farnsworth-Munsell 100-hue test can detect mild colour-vision abnormalities and contains of 84 movable tiles

**36** Regarding extraocular muscle imbalance, which of the following statements are true and which are false?
  i. The Maddox rod may be used
  ii. The Maddox wing cannot be used
  iii. The prism bar cannot be used
  iv. The slit lamp may be used
  v. The synoptophore may be used

**37** Regarding the exophthalmometer:
  i. It measures intraocular pressure
  ii. It measures the distance between the inner canthi
  iii. Reproducible measurements are difficult
  iv. Parallax can be controlled easily
  v. The edge of the exophthalmometer rests upon the lateral canthi

**38** Regarding laser modes, which of the following statements are true and which are false?
  i. Energy is delivered diffusely in Nd-YAG capsulotomy
  ii. Energy is not delivered diffusely in argon photocoagulation
  iii. Energy is maximal at the periphery of the focused laser beam
  iv. Energy focused onto the smallest spot is known as the fundamental mode
  v. Energy focused onto the smallest spot is known as the consequential mode

**39** Regarding the effect of laser, which of the following statements are true and which are false?

   i. Laser can induce ionising effects

   ii. Laser can induce thermal effects

   iii. Laser cannot induce photodisruptive effects

   iv. Laser can induce audiological effects

   v. Laser can induce scarring effects

**40** Regarding the argon blue-green laser:

   i. It emits blue (480 nm) and green (510 nm) light

   ii. It can be used to treat the outer retina

   iii. It can be used to treat the inner retina and choroid

   iv. Xanthophyll at the macula absorbs blue light

   v. A cataractous lens helps focus the laser beam

**41** Regarding Nd-YAG capsulotomy, which of the following statements are true and which are false?

   i. Endothelial damage is a recognised complication

   ii. Lens pitting is a recognised complication

   iii. Choroidal detachment is a recognised complication

   iv. Retinal detachment is a recognised complication

   v. Raised intraocular pressure is a recognised but rare complication

**42** Regarding lasers, which of the following statements are true and which are false?

   i. Argon blue-green laser is useful for retinal photocoagulation

   ii. Excimer laser is useful for corneal ablation

   iii. Nd-YAG laser is useful for phacoemulsification

   iv. Diode laser is useful for scleral breakdown

   v. Erbium: YAG laser is useful for eyelid surgery

**43** Regarding lasers, which of the following statements are true and which are false?

   i. $CO_2$ laser emits infrared radiation

   ii. Nd-YAG laser emits infrared radiation

   iii. Argon laser emits infrared radiation

   iv. Excimer laser emits infrared radiation

   v. Holmium laser emits infrared radiation

**44** Regarding side effects of fluorescein, which of the following statements are true and which are false?

   i. Anaphylaxis is a common reaction

   ii. Discolouration of urine is common

   iii. Nausea is common

   iv. Thrombophlebitis may occur

   v.  Photosensitivity reactions may occur

**45** Argon laser photocoagulation:

   i. Is never used in treatment of retinopathy of prematurity

   ii. Is used in the treatment of diabetic retinopathy

   iii. Is used in iridoplasty

   iv. Is used in capsulotomy

   v. Is used in serous retinal detachment with an optic disc pit

**46** Regarding surgical instruments:

   i. Barraquer describes a needle holder

   ii. Thornton describes a needle holder

   iii. Vectis is a device to remove the lens

   iv. Vannas is a name of scissors

   v. Westcott's is a name of scissors

**47** Regarding nucleus expression in cataract surgery:

   i. An irrigating vectis may be used

   ii. Viscoelastic may be used

   iii. Balanced salt solution (BSS) may be used

   iv. Phacoemulsification may be used

   v. A 15-degree blade may be used

**48** Regarding lasers, which of the following statements are true and which are false?

   i. The helium-neon laser emits energy with a wavelength of approximately 630 nm

   ii. Diode lasers emit energy with a wavelength of 420 nm

   iii. Argon lasers emit energy with wavelength between 620 and 650 nm

   iv. The Nd-YAG laser emits energy with wavelength between 700 and 740 nm

   v. The excimer laser emits energy with wavelength between 180 and 210 nm

**49** Regarding scanning laser polarimetry, which of the following statements are true and which are false?

    i. It measures birefringence of the retinal nerve fibre layer

    ii. It measures the density of the retinal nerve fibre layer

    iii. Laser light of 420-nm wavelength is used

    iv. Laser light of 780-nm wavelength is used

    v. Using retardation, the thickness of the retinal nerve fibre layer is measured

**50** Regarding laser safety, which of the following statements are true and which are false?

    i. Eyes may be damaged with class 1 lasers

    ii. Eyes may be damaged with class 2 lasers

    iii. Eyes may be irreversibly damaged with class 4 lasers

    iv. Class 2 lasers incorporate those in the visible spectrum

    v. Class 3 lasers typically emit 1–500 mW of energy

# 10
# Epidemiology and biostatistics

# 15 FRCOphth best-fit MCQs

1 Which of the following statistical tests is *not* affected by outliers?
   a. Standard deviation
   b. Median
   c. Mean
   d. Variance

2 In a Gaussian (normal) distribution, what percentage of the data is within 2 standard deviations of the mean?
   a. 66%
   b. 68.3%
   c. 95.5%
   d. 99.8%

3 Which of the following drivers meet the DVLA visual standards for driving a private car?
   a. 50-year-old patient with 6/6 vision both eyes, full fields but new-onset diplopia
   b. 60-year-old patient with 6/9 vision both eyes indoors but because of glare related to cataract vision deteriorates to 6/15 both eyes outdoors
   c. 40-year-old patient who lost his right eye due to trauma in childhood but has 6/9 vision in his left eye with no field defect
   d. 70-year-old patient with 6/6 vision both eyes and a bitemporal hemianopia encroaching on his central field of vision related to a pituitary adenoma

4 Which of the following drivers meet the DVLA visual standards for driving a bus?
   a. 40-year-old patient who lost his right eye due to trauma in childhood but has 6/9 vision in his left eye with no field defect in the left eye
   b. 30-year-old patient with best corrected visual acuity of 6/6 both eyes and uncorrected visual acuity of 2/60 both eyes and full fields
   c. 60-year-old patient with best corrected visual acuity of 6/9 both eyes and uncorrected visual acuity of 4/60 both eyes and full fields who is colour blind
   d. 50-year-old patient with 6/6 vision both eyes, full fields and diplopia that is controlled with patching

5  What is the approximate prevalence of blindness in developed countries?
   a. 0.01%
   b. 0.2%
   c. 1%
   d. 3%

6  Which of the following levels of evidence-based medicine should be given the most importance when assessing quality of evidence?
   a. Expert opinion
   b. Meta-analysis
   c. Case series
   d. Randomised controlled trial

7  Which of the following patients meets the criteria for severely sight-impaired registration (blind registration)?
   a. Best corrected visual acuity of 2/60 in their right eye and 6/9 in their left eye with full fields
   b. Best corrected visual acuity of 5/60 both eyes with constricted field
   c. Best corrected visual acuity of 4/60 both eyes with full field
   d. Best corrected visual acuity of 6/9 both eyes with constricted field

8  The $p$ value of a statistical test is $p < 0.05$. What does this mean?
   a. There is a 5% confidence interval
   b. 5% of the data is biased
   c. The likelihood of results occurring by chance is 5%
   d. 95% of the data is within 1 standard deviation of the mean

9  The null hypothesis for the ANCHOR study states that no difference exists between intravitreal ranibizumab and placebo sham treatment of predominantly classic choroidal neovascularisation. In fact, there is a significant difference. If the null hypothesis is accepted, what kind of error would this be?
   a. Standard error
   b. Sampling error
   c. Type I error
   d. Type II error

**10** You look back through the notes of 100 patients with suspected temporal arteritis who had a temporal artery biopsy. Ninety of these patients had elevated ESR. Seventy patients had biopsy-proven temporal arteritis which was used as the gold standard for diagnosis. Ten patients with biopsy-proven temporal arteritis did not have elevated ESR. What is the sensitivity and specificity of ESR testing for temporal arteritis in this cohort?
   a. Sensitivity 86%, specificity 33%
   b. Sensitivity 90%, specificity 10%
   c. Sensitivity 90%, specificity 70%
   d. Sensitivity 33%, specificity 90%

**11** A pharmaceutical company is developing a new topical drug for lowering intraocular pressure. They wish to assess its safety in human volunteers. After gaining permission, which phase of clinical trial will they be embarking upon?
   a. Phase 1 trial
   b. Phase 2 trial
   c. Phase 3 trial
   d. Phase 4 trial

**12** Which of the following is *not* a common error when using an exophthalmometer?
   a. Using different makes of exophthalmometer when comparing readings on separate occasions
   b. Using the same base measurement when comparing readings on separate occasions
   c. Parallax error
   d. Rounding off readings on the exopthalmometer

**13** Which of the following is an example of secondary prevention in a diabetic patient?
   a. Tight control of $HbA_{1C}$
   b. Attending diabetic retinopathy screening programme
   c. Taking a statin to control cholesterol levels
   d. Taking aspirin following a myocardial infarction

**14** Which of the following statistical tests is most appropriate to compare girls' heights with boys' heights in a school?
   **a.** Two-sample (unpaired) T-test
   **b.** Mann-Whitney U-test
   **c.** One-sample (paired) T-test
   **d.** Wilcoxon matched pairs test

**15** To assess whether and to what extent $HbA_{1C}$ relates to plasma triglyceride levels, which of the following would be the most appropriate statistical test?
   **a.** Spearman's rank correlation coefficient
   **b.** Pearson's correlation coefficient
   **c.** Fisher's exact test
   **d.** Chi-squared test

# 15 ICO true/false MCQs

**16** A random sample of 2000 normal adolescents was questioned about their use of cannabis. They were followed up 4 years later and asked about symptoms of psychosis. The probability of psychosis for non-cannabis users was 0.1, whereas the probability in cannabis users was 0.2. Regarding this study, which of the following statements are true and which are false?
  i. The relative risk of psychosis in cannabis users is 2
  ii. The absolute risk increase of psychosis in cannabis users is not relevant if the relative risk is known
  iii. The relative risk of not developing psychosis in cannabis users is the inverse of the relative risk of developing psychosis in cannabis users
  iv. The odds ratio of not developing psychosis in cannabis users is the inverse of the odds ratio of developing psychosis in cannabis users
  v. One would expect the relative risk and odds ratio to be similar in this study

**17** Regarding screening tests, which of the following statements are true and which are false?
  i. False positive describes a patient who tests positive for a disease but actually does not have it
  ii. False negative describes a patient who tests negative for a disease but actually has it
  iii. Positive predictive value is a measure of how likely someone with a positive test result is to actually have the disease
  iv. Specificity is a measure of a test's ability to identify true disease
  v. Sensitivity is a measure of a test's ability to correctly identify those without disease

**18** Which of the following definitions are true and which are false?
  i. Prevalence is the number of new cases of disease per unit population per unit time
  ii. Incidence measures the total number of cases of disease in a population at a particular point in time
  iii. Resolution refers to the smallest change that can be detected by a particular measuring device
  iv. Parametric hypotheses tests assume that the sample has an underlying distribution such as a normal distribution
  v. In a positively skewed distribution, the mean is higher than the median

**19** Regarding Estermann visual fields, which of the following statements are true and which are false?
  i. It is a test of monocular field of vision
  ii. Visual field of at least 120 degrees in the horizontal meridian must be seen to meet driving requirements
  iii. Visual field of at least 60 degrees in the vertical meridian must be seen to meet driving requirements
  iv. The target is equivalent to white Goldmann III4e settings
  v. The Estermann visual field test can be performed on a Humphrey field machine

**20** Regarding developing-world ophthalmology, which of the following statements are true and which are false?
  i. About 90% of the world's visually impaired people live in developing countries
  ii. The number of people that are visually impaired due to infectious diseases has increased in the last 20 years
  iii. Uncorrected refractive error is the commonest cause of visual impairment worldwide
  iv. 50% of all visual impairment can be prevented, treated or cured
  v. 65% of visually impaired people are under the age of 18

21 Regarding effective screening programmes, which of the following statements are true and which are false?
   i. If a patient does not attend one screening visit, they should be discharged
   ii. The screening interval should be longer than the time taken for the disease to reach an untreatable stage
   iii. Screening should be considered for a disease where early treatment is associated with better prognosis
   iv. There should be few false negatives
   v. There should be many false positives

22 Regarding assessment of effectiveness and safety of a new treatment, which of the following statements are true and which are false?
   i. The number needed to treat (NNT) is the reciprocal of the odds ratio
   ii. A drug with an NNT of 8 is highly ineffective
   iii. In therapy trials, the higher the NNT the more effective the therapy
   iv. The NNT is dependent on the baseline incidence of a disease
   v. In therapy trials, the higher the number needed to harm (NNH) the safer the therapy

23 Regarding the demonstration of a causal factor for a disease, which of the following statements are true and which are false?
   i. Demonstrating strong positive correlation is sufficient to prove causality
   ii. Elimination of the factor should reduce the risk of the disease
   iii. The causal factor should be found more frequently in the diseased than non-diseased population
   iv. Exposure to the factor should precede disease
   v. A dose-dependent relationship would be expected, i.e. increased exposure to the causative factor causes more rapid onset or more severe disease.

**24** Regarding likelihood ratios, which of the following statements are true and which are false?

   **i.** Likelihood ratio is used to assess the diagnostic accuracy of a test

   **ii.** A positive likelihood ratio of 1 indicates that the test is clinically useful

   **iii.** Likelihood ratios can be used to convert a pretest probability to a post-test probability

   **iv.** Likelihood ratios are calculated using the sensitivity and specificity of a test

   **v.** Likelihood ratios are a clinical application of Bayes' theorem

**25** Regarding confidence intervals (CI), which of the following statements are true and which are false?

   **i.** Confidence intervals reflect how well the sample data reflects the population

   **ii.** A 95% CI gives a range within which we can be 95% sure the true value lies

   **iii.** The wider the CI, the more likely that the trial result is true

   **iv.** A 95% CI is calculated as approximately 2 standard deviations either side of the trial result

   **v.** CI can be applied to non-parametric data

**26** Regarding averaging, which of the following statements are true and which are false?

   **i.** The mean is not affected by outliers

   **ii.** The mode is the sum of all the data divided by the number of data points

   **iii.** The median is higher than the mean in a negatively skewed distribution

   **i.** When there is an even number of data points, the median is the mean of the two middle numbers

   **iv.** There can only be one mode in any distribution

27 Regarding VISION 2020, which of the following statements are true and which are false?
   i. VISION 2020 is the global initiative for the elimination of avoidable blindness
   ii. Untreated refractive error causing visual impairment is an area targeted by this programme
   iii. Onchocerciasis is a disease targeted by this programme
   iv. Glaucoma is a disease targeted by this programme
   v. Non-governmental organisations (NGOs) are not part of this programme

28 Regarding childhood blindness worldwide, which of the following statements are true and which are false?
   i. It is estimated there are 1.4 million blind children in the world
   ii. Corneal scarring secondary to vitamin A deficiency or measles is common in the poorest countries
   iii. Retinopathy of prematurity is likely to become an emerging problem in middle-income countries as neonatal survival rates improve
   iv. The prevalence of refractive errors, particularly myopia, is increasing in school-age children, especially in Southeast Asia
   v. Trachoma infection and its transmission can be reduced with surgery, antibiotics, facial cleanliness and environmental change (the SAFE strategy)

29 Regarding masking in clinical trials, which of the following statements are true and which are false?
   i. In a double-masked clinical trial, neither the investigator nor the patient is aware of which intervention is being given
   ii. Masking helps to reduce publication bias
   iii. All clinical trials that are not masked are invalid
   iv. In a single-masked clinical trial, the investigator is not aware which intervention is being given but the patient is aware
   v. In a double-masked clinical trial, those interpreting the data may know which treatment a patient was given without compromising the results

**30** Regarding correlation and regression, which of the following statements are true and which are false?

    i. If variable y tends to increase as variable x increases, then there is positive correlation

    ii. Regression is the term used to describe the function (f) when looking at the following equation $y = (f)x$

    iii. The Pearson (product-moment) correlation coefficient is a numerical value which indicates the degree of scatter

    iv. The Pearson (product-moment) correlation coefficient is between −100 and +100

    v. The Spearman's rank correlation coefficient should only be used on a normally distributed data set

# 11
# Clinical genetics

# 15 FRCOphth best-fit MCQs

1  In a eukaryotic cell, the DNA-protein complex that a chromosome is comprised of is called:
   a. Chromatid
   b. Chromatin
   c. Histone
   d. Centromere

2  Which of the following does *not* play an important role in gene transcription?
   a. Promoter sequence
   b. Spliceosome
   c. Exon
   d. Ribosome

3  An inherited condition that has an earlier age of onset with each successive generation is said to show which one of the following?
   a. Penetrance
   b. Variable expressivity
   c. Anticipation
   d. Mosaicism

4  Which of the following genes is associated with age-related macular degeneration?
   a. Complement factor H gene
   b. *BEST1* gene
   c. *ABCA4* gene
   d. *RPE65* gene

5  In which of the following cases may chromosomal translocations be asymptomatic?
   a. If the translocation is balanced
   b. If the translocation is unbalanced
   c. If the translocation breakpoint passes through a gene
   d. If the translocation breakpoint passes through a gene regulatory sequence

6  In which of the following disorders is aneuploidy a feature?
   a. Myotonic dystrophy
   b. Turner's syndrome
   c. Marfan's syndrome
   d. Oculocutaneous albinism

7  Which of the following is true regarding X-linked recessive disorders?
   a. Males may be carriers
   b. Affected individuals may have affected maternal uncles
   c. Affected individuals may have affected sisters
   d. Parents of affected individuals are usually also affected

8  Which one of the following conditions is *not* inherited by mitochondrial inheritance?
   a. Leber's hereditary optic neuropathy
   b. Kearns-Sayre syndrome
   c. Chronic progressive external ophthalmoplegia
   d. Neurofibromatosis type 2

9  Which one of the following tests is used to detect ribonucleic acid (RNA)?
   a. Northern blotting
   b. Southern blotting
   c. Western blotting
   d. Eastern blotting

10 Polymerase chain reaction utilises which one of the following?
   a. DNA polymerase and two primers
   b. RNA polymerase and two primers
   c. DNA polymerase and four primers
   d. RNA polymerase and four primers

11 In mitosis the sister chromatids separate in which phase?
   a. Prophase
   b. Metaphase
   c. Anaphase
   d. Telophase

12 Which one of the following statements about ribosomes is true?
   a. They transcribe messenger RNA to build polypeptide chains
   b. They are bound to the smooth endoplasmic reticulum
   c. They freely float in the cytosol
   d. They are comprised of three subunits

13  The process of allelic frequency change entirely by chance in a population may be considered as which one of the following?
   a. Mutation
   b. Genetic drift
   c. Natural selection
   d. Gene flow

14  Which of the following is *not* used in gene therapy?
   a. Adeno-associated virus
   b. Human immunodeficiency virus 1
   c. Feline immunodeficiency virus
   d. Rhinovirus

15  Which of the following conditions is a result of trisomy?
   a. Edwards' syndrome
   b. Turner's syndrome
   c. Vogt-Koyanagi-Harada syndrome
   d. Stickler's syndrome

# 15 ICO true/false MCQs

**16** Regarding linkage analysis, which of the following are true and which are false?

   **i.** It is based on the behaviour of chromosomes at mitosis

   **ii.** Non-homologous chromosomes usually assort independently

   **iii.** The distance between two genes defined by linkage analysis is measured in centimorgans

   **iv.** The Lod score is a statistical measure of the significance of evidence for or against linkage

   **v.** Linkage analysis is useful when investigating patients with aneuploidy

**17** Regarding retinoblastoma, which of the following statements are true and which are false?

   **i.** The retinoblastoma gene is a tumour suppressor gene

   **ii.** The *RB1* (retinoblastoma) gene is on chromosome 13

   **iii.** Knudson's two-hit hypothesis applies to sporadic retinoblastoma

   **iv.** Children with heritable retinoblastoma may develop trilateral tumours

   **v.** Heritable retinoblastoma is more common than non-heritable retinoblastoma

**18** Regarding DNA polymerase:

   **i.** It assists with DNA replication

   **ii.** It acts to unwind DNA

   **iii.** It catalyses the step-wise addition of nucleotides to a primer strand that is paired to a DNA template strand

   **iv.** It joins the ends of double-stranded DNA together with a covalent bond to make a continuous DNA strand

   **v.** It requires a magnesium ion as a co-factor to function properly

**19** Regarding mutations in the *BEST1* gene, which of the following statements are true and which are false?

    i. The protein encoded by the *BEST1* gene is a calcium channel

    ii. Mutations in *BEST1* may cause autosomal recessive vitelliform macular dystrophy

    iii. Mutations in *BEST1* may cause autosomal recessive bestrophinopathy

    iv. Mutations in *BEST1* may cause autosomal dominant adult-onset macular vitelliform dystrophy

    v. Mutations in *BEST1* may cause an abnormal ERG

**20** Regarding the structure of DNA, which of the following statements are true and which are false?

    i. A nucleotide consists of a hexose sugar, phosphate group and a base

    ii. Guanine and thymine form a base pair

    iii. Adenine and thymine form a base pair

    iv. Nucleotides on the same strand of DNA are linked to each other by hydrogen bonds

    v. Complementary base pairs are linked by hydrogen bonds

**21** Regarding meiosis, which of the following statements are true and which are false?

    i. Meiosis is preceded by the $G_1$ phase of the cell cycle

    ii. Meiosis only occurs in eukaryotes

    iii. Meiosis II is similar to mitosis

    iv. Recombination of genetic material occurs in anaphase I

    v. The resultant gametes formed by meiosis are genetically identical

**22** A woman is a carrier of X-linked retinoschisis and has an unaffected partner. They wish to have children and seek genetic counselling. Which of the following statements are true and which are false?

    i. All sons will be affected with the disease

    ii. All daughters will be carriers of the disease

    iii. Half the children will be affected with the disease

    iv. Half the sons will be affected with the disease

    v. Three quarters of the children will be unaffected by the disease

**23** A woman has autosomal dominant retinitis pigmentosa and so does her partner. They wish to have children and seek genetic counselling. Which of the following statements are true and which are false?

   **i.** All the children will have the disease

   **ii.** Three quarters of the children will have the disease

   **iii.** Half the children will have the disease

   **iv.** All daughters will have the disease

   **v.** Half the children will be carriers

**24** A patient is suspected to have adenoviral conjunctivitis. Which of the following tests can be used to confirm the diagnosis?

   **i.** Restriction enzyme digestion

   **ii.** Southern blotting

   **iii.** Polymerase chain reaction (PCR)

   **iv.** Reverse transcriptase PCR

   **v.** Gram stain

**25** Regarding nonsense mutations, which of the following statements are true and which are false?

   **i.** One nucleotide is replaced by another, which changes a codon to a stop codon

   **ii.** One nucleotide is replaced by another causing a codon change, resulting in one amino acid being replaced with another

   **iii.** They may cause a frame shift

   **iv.** The resultant mRNA may be degraded

   **v.** They are likely to have no effect

**26** Regarding transcription, which of the following statements are true and which are false?

   **i.** Gene transcription is initiated by the binding of RNA polymerase to promoters

   **ii.** Gene transcription is initiated by the binding of DNA polymerase to promoters

   **iii.** Transcription factors bind to RNA

   **iv.** The TATA box is a transcription terminator

   **v.** The mRNA that is formed undergoes splicing to remove introns

**27** Which of the following methods may be used to investigate the genetics of complex disease?
  i. Adoption studies
  ii. Twin studies
  iii. Karyotyping
  iv. Association studies
  v. Restriction enzyme digestion

**28** Regarding population genetics, which of the following statements are true and which are false?
  i. An allele that causes a dominant phenotype is more common than one which causes a recessive phenotype
  ii. The Hardy-Weinberg distribution describes the relationship between genotype frequencies and gene frequencies
  iii. Heterozygote advantage may lead to a dominant allele being more common in a population
  iv. Natural selection tends to reduce the presence of a dominant mutation in the population
  v. Natural selection tends to reduce the presence of a recessive mutation in the population when it is in its heterozygous form

**29** Which of the following enzymes are required in cloning?
  i. DNA polymerase
  ii. DNA ligase
  iii. DNA helicase
  iv. Restriction endonuclease
  v. Reverse transcriptase

**30** Regarding the corneal dystrophies, which of the following are inherited in an autosomal recessive manner?
  i. Reis-Bücklers dystrophy
  ii. Lattice dystrophy type 1
  iii. Granular dystrophy
  iv. Macular dystrophy
  v. Posterior polymorphous dystrophy

# 12
# Patient investigation

# 15 FRCOphth best-fit MCQs

1   Which of the following is *not* a recognised side effect of fundus fluorescein angiography?
    **a.** Anaphylaxis
    **b.** Photosensitivity
    **c.** Vortex keratopathy
    **d.** Nausea

2   When does the choroidal (pre-arterial) phase of the fluorescein angiogram normally occur?
    **a.** 4 seconds
    **b.** 8 seconds
    **c.** 16 seconds
    **d.** 20 seconds

3   Which of the following would *not* be a contraindication to MRI orbital imaging?
    **a.** Metallic intraocular foreign body
    **b.** Ferromagnetic aneurysm clips
    **c.** Hip prosthesis
    **d.** Cardiac pacemaker

4   Which of the following parameters *cannot* be measured by A-scan ultrasonography?
    **a.** Axial length
    **b.** Lens thickness
    **c.** Intraocular tumour volume
    **d.** Anterior chamber depth

5   Which of the following optic nerve head imaging techniques measures the change in polarisation caused by the birefringence of nerve fibre layer axons?
    **a.** Optical coherence tomography (OCT)
    **b.** Glaucoma diagnosis variable corneal compensation (GDx VCC)
    **c.** Confocal scanning laser ophthalmoscope (HRT)
    **d.** Colour photography

**6** Which of the following statements best defines pattern deviation in Humphrey perimetry?
   **a.** Deviation of the patient's result from that of age-matched controls
   **b.** Deviation of the patient's result from that of age-matched controls, adjusted for a generalised depression in the overall field
   **c.** A summary of the results in a single number, principally used to monitor progression of glaucomatous damage
   **d.** The degree by which the luminance of a target is required to exceed background luminance in order to be perceived by the eye

**7** In the Snellen chart how many minutes of arc does the 6/6 letter subtend at 6 metres?
   **a.** 1 minute of arc
   **b.** 5 minutes of arc
   **c.** 6 minutes of arc
   **d.** 10 minutes of arc

**8** Which of the following blood tests does *not* have positive predictive value for temporal arteritis?
   **a.** Elevated platelet count
   **b.** Elevated erythrocyte sedimentary rate (ESR)
   **c.** Elevated eosinophil count
   **d.** Elevated C-reactive protein (CRP)

**9** A Gram stain result is called through from the pathology lab, identifying Gram-negative rods in a corneal scrape taken from a patient with probable contact lens-related microbial keratitis. Which of the following organisms is the most likely causative agent?
   **a.** *Staphylococcus aureus*
   **b.** *Pseudomonas aeruginosa*
   **c.** *Mycobacterium*
   **d.** *Acanthamoeba*

**10** Which of the following is the definition of osteoporosis on a bone mineral density scan?
   **a.** T-score within 1 standard deviation of the normal young adult value
   **b.** T-score between 1 and 2.5 standard deviations of the normal young adult value
   **c.** T-score greater than 2.5 standard deviations from the normal young adult value
   **d.** T-score greater than 3 standard deviations from the normal young adult value

11 Which of the following slit-lamp techniques is best for detecting corneal endothelial changes such as guttata?
   a. Direct illumination
   b. Scleral scatter
   c. Retroillumination
   d. Iris transillumination

12 Which of the following statements about Hess charts is most accurate?
   a. Each square on the Hess chart equals 10 degrees of arc
   b. The eye with the paretic muscle has a smaller chart compared to the other eye
   c. Stereopsis is required to complete the test
   d. A Hess chart is not useful in differentiating between a recent-onset extraocular muscle paresis and a long-standing paresis

13 A 70-year-old patient is undergoing left eye cataract surgery. The axial length of the left eye is 20.5 mm. Which of the following biometry formulas would the Royal College of Ophthalmologists guidelines recommend to choose the intraocular lens power?
   a. SRK I
   b. SRK II
   c. Hoffer Q
   d. Holladay

14 Which of the following techniques is least useful in the diagnosis of keratoconus?
   a. Slit-lamp examination
   b. Retinoscopy
   c. Gonioscopy
   d. Corneal topography

15 Which of the following statements regarding the Ziehl–Neelsen stain is most accurate?
   a. It stains *Mycobacterium tuberculosis* black
   b. It stains for acid alcohol-fast bacilli
   c. It does not stain *Nocardia* species
   d. It stains calcium deposits in band keratopathy

# 15 ICO true/false MCQs

**16** Regarding corneal imaging, which of the following statements are true and which are false?
  i. Specular microscopy allows assessment of the corneal layers at a magnification 100 times greater than slit-lamp examination
  ii. Normal endothelial cell density is 3000 cells/mm$^2$
  iii. A patient with a preoperative endothelial cell count of 500 cells/mm$^2$ is at significant risk of corneal decompensation
  iv. In corneal topography, steep curvatures are represented by cold colours (e.g. blue and green)
  v. In corneal topography, flat curvatures are represented by warm colours (e.g. yellow and red)

**17** Regarding indocyanine green (ICG) angiography, which of the following statements are true and which are false?
  i. About 98% of ICG molecules bind to serum proteins
  ii. ICG angiography is useful in delineating the choroidal circulation
  iii. ICG should not be given to patients with known iodine allergy
  iv. ICG emission is in the near-infrared spectrum
  v. ICG angiography is contraindicated in pregnancy

**18** Regarding magnetic resonance imaging (MRI), which of the following statements are true and which are false?
  i. MRI exposes a patient to ionising radiation
  ii. In $T_1$-weighted images vitreous is hypointense (black) and fat is hyperintense (white)
  iii. In $T_1$-weighted images bone appears hypointense (black)
  iv. The bright signal of orbital fat on conventional $T_1$-weighted images frequently obscures other orbital contents
  v. Gadolinium enhances $T_2$-weighted images

**19** Regarding computed tomography (CT), which of the following statements are true and which are false?

i. CT is contraindicated in patients with suspected metallic intraocular foreign bodies

ii. CT exposes patients to ionising radiation

iii. CT is the investigation of choice for imaging soft tissue injuries

iv. CT is better tolerated than MRI scanning by claustrophobic patients

v. Dense structures appear white on CT scans

**20** Regarding optical coherence tomography (OCT), which of the following statements are true and which are false?

i. OCT is analogous to B-scan ultrasonography but uses light instead of sound

ii. OCT requires clear media

iii. Fourier-domain OCT allows faster image acquisition than time-domain OCT

iv. Time-domain OCT has less motion artefact than Fourier-domain OCT

v. Time-domain OCT has axial resolution of less than 10 microns

**21** Regarding perimetry, which of the following statements are true and which are false?

i. The Goldmann perimeter is a form of kinetic perimetry

ii. The Humphrey perimeter is a form of kinetic perimetry

iii. The 24-2 strategy on Humphrey perimetry tests 24 points

iv. The Swedish Interactive Thresholding Algorithm (SITA) program allows data to be acquired more quickly than standard full-threshold programs

v. The greyscale printout in individuals with high false negative responses may produce a clover-leaf pattern

**22** Regarding electroretinography (ERG), which of the following statements are true and which are false?

i. The cone response can be isolated by using a flickering light stimulus at 10 Hz

ii. The cone response can be isolated by using a flickering light stimulus at 30 Hz

iii. The cone response can be isolated by using a flickering light stimulus at 60 Hz

iv. Isolated rod responses generate large a-wave components

v. Blue light can be used to isolate rod responses

**23** Regarding electrooculography (EOG), which of the following statements are true and which are false?

   i. The Arden ratio is calculated by dividing the light peak by the dark trough

   ii. EOG measures activity of the optic nerve

   iii. An Arden ratio of 1 is normal

   iv. The absolute amplitude of EOG responses is similar across a population of normal subjects

   v. The EOG is subnormal in juvenile Best's macular dystrophy

**24** Regarding visual evoked potentials (VEP), which of the following statements are true and which are false?

   i. VEP is a recording of electrical activity of the visual cortex created by stimulation of the retina

   ii. VEP can be used to assess visual function in babies

   iii. VEP can be used to assess the extent of traumatic optic neuropathy

   iv. In albinism, VEP studies can demonstrate less crossed nerve fibres at the optic chiasm than normal

   v. VEP can be used as an objective assessment of visual function in suspected functional visual loss

**25** Regarding thyroid function tests, which of the following statements are true and which are false?

   i. In primary hypothyroidism, thyroid stimulating hormone (TSH) levels are suppressed

   ii. Systemically ill patients can have a temporary decrease in thyroid hormone and TSH levels

   iii. Thyroid function tests in patients on phenytoin should be interpreted with caution

   iv. Thyroid eye disease cannot develop in euthyroid patients

   v. In Graves' disease, serum IgG antibodies bind to the TSH receptor stimulating thyroid hormone production

**26** Regarding acid-base balance, which of the following statements are true and which are false?

   i. Respiratory alkalosis would be expected in a patient who was hyperventilating

   ii. Oral acetazolamide treatment can lead to metabolic acidosis

   iii. Diabetic ketoacidosis causes a respiratory acidosis

   iv. Vomiting is a cause of metabolic alkalosis

   v. Guillain-Barré syndrome can be associated with respiratory acidosis

**27** Regarding urinanalysis, which of the following statements are true and which are false?

  i. Lying flat increases urinary protein output
  ii. Exercise increases urinary protein output
  iii. Microalbuminuria refers to urinary levels of albumin with reduced molecular weight compared to normal
  iv. The presence of a small amount of glucose in the urine is common
  v. Detecting blood in urine always indicates pathology

**28** Regarding HLA antigens, which of the following statements are true and which are false?

  i. The major histocompatibility complex (MHC) codes for molecules known as human leucocyte antigens (HLA)
  ii. The MHC cluster of genes is located on the X chromosome
  iii. HLA tissue typing reduces the risk of graft rejection
  iv. HLA-B27 is associated with acute anterior uveitis
  v. HLA antigens are expressed on all cells of the body

**29** Regarding cover testing, which of the following statements are true and which are false?

  i. The cover/uncover test identifies manifest deviations
  ii. The alternate cover test identifies the sum of latent and manifest deviations
  iii. The cover/uncover test is a dissociative test
  iv. The prism cover test can only be used to assess horizontal squints
  v. Dissociated vertical deviations can be detected on cover testing

**30** Regarding cardiac enzymes associated with myocardial infarction (MI), which of the following statements are true and which are false?

  i. Elevated troponin T levels are selective for cardiac injury
  ii. Elevated lactate dehydrogenase (LDH) levels are selective for cardiac injury
  iii. Elevated creatinine kinase (CK) levels are selective for cardiac injury
  iv. LDH levels remain elevated for up to 10 days following MI
  v. Troponin T is released into the serum 1 hour following MI

# Answers

# 1. Anatomy FRCOphth answers

**1    C**    The cranial nerves supply a number of different structures within the head and neck region. The oculomotor nerve supplies the superior, medial and inferior rectus along with the inferior oblique and levator palpebrae superioris. The abducens or 4th cranial nerve supplies the lateral rectus. The facial (7th) cranial nerve supplies the muscles of facial expression as well as the stapedius muscle, stylohyoid and posterior belly of the digastric muscle. The glossopharyngeal, or 9th cranial nerve, supplies parasympathetic fibres to the parotid gland, via the otic ganglion, and motor fibres to the stylopharyngeus muscle.[1]
**Difficulty level: 3**

**2    A**    The medial wall of the orbit is long and slender, measuring approximately 0.2–0.4 mm in thickness. The medial wall is formed by the frontal processes of the maxilla, the lacrimal bone, orbital plate of the ethmoid and also the body of the sphenoid. The lateral wall of the orbital wall is formed by the orbital surfaces of the greater wing of sphenoid posteriorly and zygomatic bone more anteriorly. The roof of the orbit is formed by the lesser wing of sphenoid and orbital plate of the frontal bone. The floor of the orbit is formed by the orbital part of the maxilla, orbital surface of the zygoma and a portion of the palatine bone.[1]
**Difficulty level: 4**

**3    B**    The levator palpebrae superioris (LPS) is supplied by the superior branch of the oculomotor nerve, and this branch also supplies the superior rectus. The trochlear or 4th cranial nerve supplies the superior oblique muscle. The trigeminal nerve is divided into ophthalmic, maxillary and mandibular branches. The maxillary branch passes through the foramen rotundum and subsequently passes through the inferior orbital fissure. It eventually forms a number of cutaneous branches that supply the lower eyelid, nose, upper lip and cheek. The mandibular branch supplies the muscles of mastication.[1]
**Difficulty level: 3**

**4    C**    The approximate volume of the orbit is 30 ml. This is of relevance regarding orbital surgery, for example with exenteration and evisceration.

The orbit is pyramidal in shape, with its apex directed posteriorly. The medial and lateral walls of the orbit are approximately 45 degrees to each other. The orbital axis is approximately 22 degrees to the sagittal plane. Inflammatory conditions that may affect the entire orbit include Wegener's granulomatosis, thyroid eye disease and orbital pseudotumor. Orbital decompression surgery involves creating more space in the orbit and indications can include exposure keratopathy secondary to orbital pathology, compressive optic neuropathy and orbital congestion.[1,2]
**Difficulty level: 3**

5   **D**   The medial rectus insertion lies 5.5 mm from the limbus, the inferior rectus 6.5 mm, the lateral rectus 6.9 mm and the superior rectus 7.7 mm from the limbus. The origin of insertion is known as the spiral of Tillaux. The longest muscle is the superior rectus, and the lateral rectus has the longest tendon length at 8.4 mm. The insertion points of muscles are of importance in strabismus surgery and are checked during a procedure. Usually, in muscle resection surgery the muscle is sutured to the stump of the incised muscle, and in recession surgery the muscle is sutured to the insertion using a 'hang-back' or guarded 'hang-back' technique.[1]
**Difficulty level: 3**

6   **C**   The inferior oblique muscle is innervated by the oculomotor nerve. Its primary action is extorsion of the eye, its secondary action is elevation and tertiary action is abduction. Maximal inferior oblique action is in the adducted position.[1]
**Difficulty level: 2**

7   **A**   The limbus has multiple functions, including supplying nutrients to the peripheral cornea, hypersensitivity responses and immunosurveillance of the ocular surface. Stem cells are also present here. The anatomical limbus is bordered anteriorly by a connecting line between Bowman's and the end of Descemet's line. Other important changes occur at the level of the limbus, including regular to irregular collagen rearrangement consistent with the beginning of the sclera. Pathologists define the limbus as a block of tissue bordered anteriorly by a line passing through the termination of Schwalbe's line and the junction of the conjunctival and corneal epithelium.[1]
**Difficulty level: 4**

8   **D**   The oculomotor, abducens and nasociliary nerve pass within the common tendinous ring. The four extraocular recti muscles also originate from

a common tendinous ring, although they also possess fibrous bands with specific attachments to the orbital walls throughout their course.[1]

**Difficulty level: 2**

9　**D**　The foramen ovale pierces through the greater wing of sphenoid and transmits the mandibular nerve, accessory meningeal artery and infrequently the lesser petrosal nerve. The foramen of Magendie is an opening from the fourth ventricle. The foramen lacerum transmits the internal carotid artery and some sympathetic nerves. The foramen rotundum, as well as transmitting the maxillary nerve, also transmits small veins from the cavernous sinus.[1]

**Difficulty level: 3**

10　**A**　The lacrimal gland receives its sensory input from the ophthalmic nerve via the trigeminal ganglion. Its sympathetic supply is via the deep petrosal nerve and this passes through the pterygopalatine ganglion. The parasympathetic nerve supply is from the lacrimal nucleus situated in the inferior part of the pons, and the fibres are transmitted through the nervus intermedius.[1]

**Difficulty level: 4**

11　**C**　The pretarsal portion of the eyelid derives its arterial supply from the superficial temporal artery. It also receives some branches from the facial arteries. The post-tarsal portion of the eyelid is derived from branches of the ophthalmic artery. Venous drainage is via a series of anastomoses to the ophthalmic veins and eventually on to the cavernous sinus.[1]

**Difficulty level: 3**

12　**D**　The superior oblique originates from the area superomedial to the optic canal and its tendon runs approximately 10 mm before winding around the trochlea. The length of the muscle belly is 32 mm and it is the only muscle to form a fusiform shape. The trochlear (IV) cranial nerve inserts into the upper border of the muscle.[1]

**Difficulty level: 5**

13　**B**　The suspensory ligament of Lockwood is a thickened connective tissue band between the inferior oblique and inferior rectus. Müller's muscle sits inferiorly to the levator palepbrae superioris. The accessory glands of Wolfring lie inferiorly to the palpebral conjunctiva.[1]

**Difficulty level: 3**

**14 B** The caruncula lacrimalis is a small mound of highly vascular tissue lying in the medial aspect of the eye, lateral to the inner canthus. Tears are drained from the medial aspect of the conjunctival sac, through the lacrimal puncta, which are within two small swellings known as the papillae lacrimalis.[1]
**Difficulty level: 3**

**15 A** Terminal branches of the ophthalmic artery are the dorsal nasal and supratrochlear branches. The lacrimal and zygomaticofacial arteries are earlier branches of the ophthalmic artery.[1]
**Difficulty level: 4**

**16 A** The intraocular portion of the optic nerve is supplied by scleral vessels which are known as the circle of Zinn-Haller, as well as central retinal arterial vessels, choroidal vessels and pial blood vessels. Retinal arterioles supply retinal layers.[1]
**Difficulty level: 3**

**17 D** The superior orbital fissure transmits the abducens, trochlear and oculomotor nerves, as well as the superior ophthalmic vein. Within the common tendinous ring, the optic nerve and ophthalmic artery are present.[1]
**Difficulty level: 2**

**18 C** The canal of Schlemm runs around the eye at the corneoscleral junction. It is lined with endothelium. There is no direct communication with the passages of the trabecular meshwork – they are separated by the endothelium lining the canal, connective tissue and endothelium lining the trabecular meshwork. The canal is drained by collector channels which join the deep scleral venous plexus, which eventually drain into the anterior ciliary veins.[1]
**Difficulty level: 4**

**19 D** The iris consists of stroma anteriorly (derived from mesenchyme) and two epithelial layers posteriorly (derived from neural ectoderm). The cells of the posterior epithelial layer contain melanin and are continuous with the inner non-pigmented ciliary epithelium. The anterior iris surface is divided into a central pupillary zone and peripheral ciliary zone, demarcated by the collarette where the iris is thickest.[1]
**Difficulty level: 4**

**20** **A** The dilator pupillae muscle is innervated by sympathetic fibres via the long ciliary nerves.[1]
**Difficulty level: 4**

**21** **B** The posterior lens surface is more convex than the anterior. The lens capsule is an elastic basement membrane formed by the lens epithelium anteriorly and the superficial lens fibres posteriorly. It is thickest at the equator and thinnest at the poles. The lens epithelium differentiates into lens fibres which have a hexagonal cross section.[1]
**Difficulty level: 4**

**22** **A** During accommodation, contraction of the meridional ciliary muscle fibres pulls the ciliary body forwards and contraction of the circular ciliary muscle fibres pulls the ciliary body inwards. The tension on the zonules is reduced and the lens acquires a more globular shape.[1]
**Difficulty level: 3**

**23** **C** The ciliary body is on average 6 mm wide and consists of a ridged anterior part (pars plicata) which is continuous with the periphery of the iris. The smooth posterior part (pars plana) is continuous with the choroid. The ciliary processes arise from the pars plicata and the zonules attach in between these.[1]
**Difficulty level: 4**

**24** **B** The non-pigmented ciliary epithelium is the inner layer and is the anterior continuation of the neural retina. The pigmented epithelium forms the outer layer and is the continuation of the retinal pigment epithelium. The non-pigmented cells contain Golgi apparatus, endoplasmic reticulum and mitochondria, whereas the pigmented cells contain numerous melanosomes, Golgi apparatus and mitochondria. Both layers produce aqueous humour.[1]
**Difficulty level: 4**

**25** **D** The external layer of the choroid consists of connective tissue containing melanocytes and vessels including branches of the short posterior ciliary arteries. The capillaries of the middle layer are lined with fenestrated endothelium (and not epithelium). Bruch's membrane consists of five components, one of which is the basement membrane of the RPE.[1]
**Difficulty level: 4**

**26** **D** The neurosensory retina is comprised of 10 layers, of which the outer nuclear layer consists of nuclei of rod and cone cells. The inner plexiform

layer consists of synaptic connections between bipolar, amacrine and ganglion cells. The nerve fibre layer consists of axons of ganglion cells.[1]
**Difficulty level: 4**

27 **C**  The nerve fibres anterior to the disc are non-myelinated, whereas those posterior to the disc are myelinated. The optic nerve passes through the optic canal, which is in the lesser wing of sphenoid. The arterial supply of the orbital part of the nerve is from the central retinal artery and posterior ciliary arteries.[1]
**Difficulty level: 4**

28 **A**  The two parietal bones articulate with each other at the sagittal suture. The parietal bone articulates with the occipital bone at the lamboid suture. The temporal suture does not exist.[1]
**Difficulty level: 3**

29 **D**  The endosteal layer of the dura mater does not extend through the foramen magnum. It is the meningeal layer of the dura mater that is continuous with the spinal cord. The dural fold called the falx cerebri is attached to the crista galli. The tentorium cerebelli covers the upper surface of the cerebellum and supports the occipital lobes. The subdural space separates the dura and arachnoid mater; the subarachnoid space separates the arachnoid and pia mater.[1]
**Difficulty level: 4**

30 **A**  The sella turcica is bounded posteriorly by the dorsum sellae. The sphenoidal sinuses lie inferiorly to the pituitary gland. The pituitary gland lies inferiorly to the optic chiasm, and so pituitary lesions compress the optic chiasm from below, causing a bitemporal field defect that is often denser superiorly than inferiorly.[1]
**Difficulty level: 2**

31 **C**  The ophthalmic artery runs through the optic canal. The maxillary nerve runs through the foramen rotundum. The vagus nerve runs through the jugular foramen.[1]
**Difficulty level: 4**

32 **D**  Cranial nerves III, IV and Va run in the lateral wall of the cavernous sinus (Vb passes inferiorly). The abducens nerve (VI) and the internal carotid artery pass forwards through the sinus. The optic nerve does not pass in the cavernous sinus.[1]
**Difficulty level: 4**

**33 A** Lesions of the cerebellopontine angle may compress the trigeminal nerve (causing loss of corneal reflex), facial and vestibulocochlear nerves and more rarely other lower cranial nerves. Acoustic neuromas are a common lesion in this area. The oculomotor nerve does not run through this region.[1]
**Difficulty level: 4**

**34 D** The vagus nerve innervates the muscles of the palate, pharynx and larynx that contract in the gag reflex, during swallowing and in the cough reflex. The vagus nerve promotes peristalsis in the small intestine. The vagus nerve does not innervate salivary glands.[3]
**Difficulty level: 3**

**35 C** The cerebellum comprises two lateral hemispheres separated by the midline vermis. The most anterior and caudal part of the lateral lobe is the flocculus, attached to a nodule in the midline. Together they form the flocculonodular lobe, an important part of the vestibular system. The bulge of the lateral lobe which projects inferiorly posterolateral to the medulla is the tonsil. It is implicated in 'coning' (compression of the medulla oblongata secondary to raised intracranial pressure). The cerebellum is linked to the brainstem by three pairs of cerebellar peduncles. The superior peduncle connects to the midbrain, the middle peduncle to the pons and the inferior peduncle to the medulla. The inferior cerebellar peduncle carries fibres linking the vestibular nuclei, spinal cord and inferior olivary nuclei to the cerebellum.[3]
**Difficulty level: 4**

**36 C** Two types of afferent fibres enter the cerebellar cortex. Climbing fibres originate in the contralateral inferior olivary nucleus. All other cerebellar afferents enter as mossy fibres and terminate in the granular layer. One type of efferent, Purkinje cells, convey information to the deep cerebellar nuclei.[3]
**Difficulty level: 3**

**37 C** About 30% of the primary visual cortex represents the macula.[3]
**Difficulty level: 2**

**38 D** The frontal, maxillary, anterior and middle groups of the ethmoidal sinus drain into the middle meatus of the nose. The posterior group of the ethmoidal sinus, which lie close to the optic canal, open into the superior meatus of the nose. The sphenoidal sinus opens into the nasal cavity into the sphenoethmoidal recess above the superior concha.[4]

**Difficulty level: 3**

39  **A**  The pulmonary artery originates from the right ventricle. The pulmonary vein drains into the left atrium. The left ventricle pumps this oxygenated blood to the body via the aorta. Deoxygenated blood re-enters the heart via the right atrium.[5]

**Difficulty level: 1**

40  **B**  Arteries do not contain valves to prevent backflow. Venous valves break up columns of blood, thus relieving the more dependent parts of excessive pressure, and allowing venous blood to only flow towards the heart.[5]

**Difficulty level: 1**

41  **D**  Lymphatic vessels and nodes are not present in the orbit. Lymphatic drainage of the eyelids and conjunctiva parallels the course of veins. Submandibular lymph nodes drain the medial aspect of periocular tissue. Superficial preauricular lymph nodes drain the lateral aspect of periocular tissue.[4]

**Difficulty level: 3**

42  **B**  The thoracic duct drains lymph from most of the body, except the right side of the head and neck, the right upper limb and the right side of the thorax, which drain through the right lymphatic duct.[5]

**Difficulty level: 3**

43  **C**  The lateral geniculate nucleus contains six layers of grey matter. Layers 1, 4 and 6 receive input from the contralateral optic nerve and layers 2, 3 and 5 receive input from the ipsilateral optic nerve.[4]

**Difficulty level: 3**

44  **A**  The lateral geniculate nuclei are supplied by a double blood supply from the anterior choroidal and posterior cerebral arteries.[4]

**Difficulty level: 4**

45  **C**  The ophthalmic division of the trigeminal nerve runs in the lateral wall of the cavernous sinus. The maxillary division lies inferiorly in the cavernous sinus, exiting via the foramen rotundum. The mandibular division does not enter the cavernous sinus.[4]

**Difficulty level: 2**

**46 B**   The frontal, trochlear and lacrimal nerves pass through the superior orbital fissure and outside the annulus of Zinn. The oculomotor, abducens and nasociliary nerves pass inside the annulus of Zinn.[4]
**Difficulty level: 2**

**47 A**   The two lobes of the lacrimal gland are divided by the lateral extent of the levator aponeurosis.[4]
**Difficulty level: 3**

**48 B**   Cranial nerve IV has the longest intracranial course and is the most commonly injured nerve during head injury. Cranial nerve VI can also be injured. Raised intracranial pressure is most likely to damage cranial nerve VI.[4]
**Difficulty level: 2**

**49 D**   A homonymous visual field defect must be caused by a lesion posterior to the chiasm. Inferior fibres running in the temporal lobe map the superior visual field.[3]
**Difficulty level: 2**

**50 A**   A lesion in the left optic tract would cause a right homonymous hemianopia.[3]
**Difficulty level: 2**

## References

1 Forrester J, Dick A, McMenamin A, *et al. The Eye: basic sciences in practice*. 2nd ed. Philadelphia: Saunders Elsevier; 2007. (**q1**) pp. 68–77, (**q2**) pp. 3–6, (**q3, q4**) pp. 67–70, (**q5**) pp. 64–5, (**q6**) pp. 59–62, (**q7**) p. 62, (**q8**) pp. 62–3, (**q9**) p. 11, (**q10**) pp. 85–7, (**q11**) p. 80, (**q12**) pp. 64–5, (**q13**) pp. 80–1, (**q14**) pp. 85–7, (**q15**) pp. 80–1, (**q16**) pp. 58–60, (**q17**) p. 6, (**q18**) pp. 21–4, (**q19**) pp. 26–8, (**q20**) p. 28, (**q21, q23**) pp. 31–3, (**q22**) p. 33, (**q24**) pp. 38–44, (**q25**) pp. 40–4, (**q26**) pp. 39–44, (**q27**) pp. 56–8, (**q28**) pp. 5–8, (**q29**) pp. 5–10, (**q30**) pp. 4–9, (**q31**) pp. 5–11, (**q32**) pp. 6–11, (**q33**) pp. 3–9.

2 Wong TW. *The Ophthalmological Examinations Review*. Singapore: World Scientific Publishing Co; 2007. (**q4**) p. 290.

3 Crossman A, Neary D. *Neuroanatomy – an illustrated colour text*. 2nd ed. Edinburgh: Churchill Livingstone; 2000. (**q34**) p. 115, (**q35, q36**) pp. 120–4, (**q37**) p. 164, (**q49, q50**) p. 165.

4 Snell R, Lemp M. *Clinical Anatomy of the Eye*. 2nd ed. Malden: Blackwell Publishing; 2006. (**q38**) pp. 79–86, (**q41**) p. 102, (**q43**) p. 397, (**q44**) p. 389, (**q45**) pp. 313–21, (**q46**) p. 64, (**q47**) p. 114, (**q48**) pp. 310–11.

5 Moore K, Dalley A. *Clinically Orientated Anatomy*. 4th ed. Philadelphia: Lippincott, Williams & Wilkins; 1999. (**q39**) p. 120, (**q40**) p. 32, (**q42**) p. 1062.

# 1. Anatomy ICO answers

**51**   i. T      ii. F      iii. T      iv. F      v. T

The cranial vault consists of eight bones, of which two are paired. The facial skeleton has a total of 14 bones, of which only two are single. The cranium contains a number of cavities such as the cranial, orbital, nasal and oral cavities. The nasal cavity is concerned with respiration and olfaction principally. The cranial cavity supports the brain, and the orbital cavity contains space for the orbits and adnexae. The largest bone in the skull is the parietal bone, and posterior to this is the occipital bone.[1]

**Difficulty level: 2**

**52**   i. F      ii. T      iii. F      iv. F      v. T

The sinuses principally act to warm and moisten air, add resonance to the voice and also lighten the skull. They tend not to act to cool the brain. The frontal sinus is supplied by the supraorbital nerve, which explains the referred pain in frontal sinusitis. The maxillary sinus is in contact with the middle meatus of the nasal cavity via an aperture which empties into the lower part of the hiatus semilunaris. Of note, the opening is relatively high up on the maxillary sinus wall and so does not permit drainage in the upright position.[1]

**Difficulty level: 2**

**53**   i. T      ii. F      iii. T      iv. F      v. T

The medial rectus inserts approximately 5.5 mm from the limbus, with the lateral rectus inserting approximately 7.0 mm from the limbus. The superior rectus has the longest muscle belly length of all of the extraocular muscles, and the superior oblique tendon is the longest tendon, winding around the trochlea. The inferior oblique muscle has the shortest tendon, and its muscle fibres almost reach the posterolateral quadrant of the sclera where the muscle inserts.[1]

**Difficulty level: 2**

**54**    i. T      ii. F      iii. T      iv. F      v. T

The origin of the trochlear nerve lies at the level of the inferior colliculus, from the anterior part of the aqueductal grey matter. The fibres first past anteriorly and laterally, before passing posteriorly around the periaqueductal grey matter. The abducens nerve origin lies in the midpons, and the fibres pass anteriorly first to emerge on the lower border of the pons. Embryologically, the ophthalmic division of the trigeminal nerve represents the nerve to the frontonasal swelling. The maxillary branch of the trigeminal nerve passes through the foramen rotundum and then traverses the pterygopalatine fossa. Hutchinson's sign, vesicles on the tip of the nose, imply nasociliary nerve involvement in herpes zoster ophthalmicus.[1]

**Difficulty level: 3**

**55**    i. F      ii. T      iii. F      iv. F      v. T

The lacrimal canaliculi are of 10 mm length approximately (0.5 mm diameter), and both the superior and inferior canaliculi have both horizontal and vertical components. These unite to form the common canaliculus, which drains into the lacrimal sac. The lacrimal gland, approximately 20 mm in length, is divided into two segments: a larger, orbital part, and a smaller palpebral section. The orbital part is lodged in the lacrimal fossa. The blood supply to the lacrimal gland is via the lacrimal artery, and venous drainage occurs via the ophthalmic veins. Lymphatic drainage of the lacrimal gland is through the preauricular lymph node.[1]

**Difficulty level: 3**

**56**    i. T      ii. F      iii. F      iv. T      v. F

The optic chiasm is essential for binocular vision, with nerve fibres from the nasal hemiretina crossing over on each side. The fibres emanating from the temporal hemiretina do not cross in the chiasm. It is situated at the junction of the anterior wall and the floor of the third ventricle. It lies behind the optic groove. The tuber cinereum lies behind and below the chiasm between the mammillary bodies. The lateral geniculate nucleus (LGN) consists of six laminae orientated in a dome-shaped mound. The geniculocalcarine tracts wind in varying degrees around the tip of the lateral ventricle. The lateral root is larger and the medial root smaller.[1]

**Difficulty level: 3**

**57**  **i.** F     **ii.** F     **iii.** F     **iv.** F     **v.** F

The corneal endothelium consists of simple squamous cells, arranged in hexagonal morphology over the posterior surface of the cornea. The cells sit on Descemet's membrane and are metabolically very active. As a consequence of this, they possess large numbers of mitochondria. There are approximately 350 000 cells/mm$^3$ per cornea, and cell density usually decreases with increasing age. Damage to corneal endothelial cells and a density below 1500/mm$^3$ usually leads to corneal oedema. Excrescences, known as Hassall-Henle bodies, are present in Fuchs' endothelial dystrophy.[1]

**Difficulty level: 4**

**58**  **i.** T     **ii.** F     **iii.** T     **iv.** F     **v.** T

The retina consists of two principle layers – an inner neurosensory layer and outer retinal pigment epithelial (RPE) layer. The neural retina is firmly attached at the ora serrata and the margins of the optic nerve head. The order of the layers discussed in the question are (from out to in): choriocapillaris, Bruch's membrane, retinal pigment epithelial layer, outer nuclear layer, outer plexiform layer, inner nuclear layer, inner plexiform layer, ganglion cell layer and finally the nerve fibre layer.[1]

**Difficulty level: 3**

**59**  **i.** F     **ii.** F     **iii.** T     **iv.** T     **v.** F

The blood supply to the orbit principally consists of the ophthalmic artery, from which the central retinal artery originates. It does not originate from the lacrimal artery. The retina is nourished by both the central retinal artery, and for the outer third, the choroidal circulation. There are a number of important sites around the orbit involving anastomoses of branches of the internal and external carotid arteries. An example is that between the transverse facial artery and the lacrimal artery. This is important clinically as it may form a potential route for the spread of infection. The ophthalmic artery does not divide into infratrochlear and nasal branches.[1]

**Difficulty level: 3**

**60**   i. T      ii. F      iii. F      iv. T      v. T

The retina is a highly metabolically active tissue in the human body, higher than any other tissue by weight. The retina has a very selective blood-tissue barrier, rather like the brain. It has a double blood supply – the inner two thirds are nourished from the central retinal vessels, whereas the outer third receives its vascular supply from the choroidal circulation. The central retinal artery arises from the ophthalmic artery in the optic canal and passes through the subarachnoid space that surrounds the optic nerve. As it passes forwards it does so with the central retinal vein.[1]

**Difficulty level: 2**

**61**   i. T      ii. F      iii. F      iv. T      v. F

The optic nerve is the only central nervous system tract that can be directly visualised by the clinician. It can be divided into four main sections: intraocular (approximately 1 mm in length), orbital (approximately 25–30 mm in length), intracanalicular (4–10 mm) and intracranial (10 mm). The intraocular portion of the nerve fibres are not myelinated, and are damaged in glaucoma. The absence of retinal tissue at the optic disc is responsible for the blind spot.[1]

**Difficulty level: 3**

**62**   i. F      ii. T      iii. F      iv. F      v. T

The retinal pigment epithelium has an active pumping mechanism and a large number of mitochondria are present. Lysosomes are present in high concentrations to degrade photoreceptor disks. Both smooth and rough endoplasmic reticula are present for protein and lipid synthesis. Apical microvilli are essential for adhesion and also phagocytosis. In order to maintain the blood-retinal barrier the cells have large junctional complexes to promote cell adhesion.[1]

**Difficulty level: 4**

**63**   i. F      ii. T      iii. T      iv. F      v. F

Schlemm's canal is a circumferential channel lined by endothelium. The canal sits on the outer aspect of the trabecular meshwork. It is drained by 25–30 collector channels and between two and eight aqueous veins. Schwalbe's line lies anteriorly to the apex of the trabecular meshwork. Aqueous humour passes both through the inter- and intratrabecular spaces. The scleral spur forms the base of the trabecular meshwork, which consists of three subdivided zones. A resistance to aqueous outflow is thought to be one mechanism that may result in glaucoma. This may arise from additional extracellular matrix deposition, causing an increase in intraocular pressure.[1]

**Difficulty level: 5**

**64**   i. T      ii. F      iii. T      iv. F      v. F

Rods contain the visual pigment rhodopsin, and are long and slender cells compared to cones, which are shorter and more conical. Rods are phagocytosed by RPE in a circadian manner. Cones are tightly packed and are exclusive to the foveal region of the retina. Cones have an outer segment which is connected to the mitochondria-rich inner segment. Cones are connected by an inner fibre to spherules which synapse to bipolar and horizontal cells. A single cone may be connected to up to six horizontal cells in the immediate vicinity. Cone lamellae, or discs, are not surrounded by a plasma membrane.[1]

**Difficulty level: 3**

**65**   i. F      ii. T      iii. F      iv. F      v. F

The oculomotor nerve, the third cranial nerve, innervates many extraocular muscles and originates at the level of the superior colliculus. The Edinger-Westphal nucleus contains small parasympathetic neurones. The nerve extends forwards and downwards into the interpeduncular fossa lateral to the posterior communicating artery. It passes between the superior cerebellar artery and the posterior cerebral artery. The nerve runs in the upper lateral wall of the cavernous sinus and enters the orbit through the superior orbital fissure.[1]

**Difficulty level: 3**

**66**   i. T      ii. T      iii. T      iv. T      v. T

The corneal epithelium forms the sensory receptor for the corneal reflex, and the afferent pathway for this reflex is the long ciliary and nasolacrimal nerves. The efferent pathway is carried by the temporal and zygomatic nerves of the facial nerve, and the effector muscle is the orbicularis oculi. The retinal cones form the receptors for the blinking to bright light reflex, and for the loud noise reflex, the afferent pathway is the vestibulocochlear nerve, with the efferent pathway being the temporal and zygomatic branches of the facial nerve, and the effector muscle is orbicularis oculi.[1]

**Difficulty level: 4**

**67**  i. F  ii. F  iii. T  iv. F  v. T

The oculomotor cranial nerve supplies the majority of extraocular muscles in the eye. It innervates the medial, inferior and superior rectus as well as the inferior oblique. The superior branch of the oculomotor nerve supplies the levator palpebrae superioris. The abducens (6th) cranial nerve supplies the lateral rectus, whereas the superior oblique is innervated by the trochlear (4th) nerve. Occasionally, following a cranial nerve palsy, abberant regeneration occurs resulting in different cranial nerves supplying different muscles than usual. This can result in a narrowing of the palpebral aperture on lateral gaze when the patient is examined clinically.[1]

**Difficulty level: 2**

**68**  i. T  ii. T  iii. F  iv. F  v. T

The roof of the orbit is formed by a small portion of the lesser wing of the sphenoid and the frontal bone. The lateral wall is formed by the zygomatic bone and the greater wing of sphenoid bone posteriorly. The medial wall is formed by the lacrimal bone, the orbital plate of the ethmoid, the frontal process of the maxilla and the sphenoid bone. The floor of the orbit is formed by the zygoma, the orbital plate of the maxilla, and the palatine bone. The orbital cavities are separated from each other by ethmoidal and sphenoidal sinuses, as well as the nasal cavity.[1]

**Difficulty level: 3**

**69**  i. F  ii. F  iii. T  iv. T  v. T

The middle cranial fossa contains a number of foramina, as well as a hollow forming the optic canal and the superior orbital fissure. The foramen ovale transmits the accessory meningeal artery and the mandibular nerve. The foramen spinosum, posterolateral to the foramen ovale, transmits the middle meningeal artery and the vein. The foramen lacerum, located at the apex of the petrous temporal bone, transmits the internal carotid artery, as well as sympathetic nerves and a small plexus of veins. The foramen rotundum transmits the maxillary nerve and small veins from the cavernous sinus.[1]

**Difficulty level: 4**

**70**   i. F      ii. F      iii. T      iv. F      v. F

The iris, ciliary body and choroid constitute the uveal tract, and this is bordered anteriorly by the pupillary margin and posteriorly by the optic disc. The iris is approximately 12 mm in diameter, and the pupil may vary from 1–8 mm in diameter. The iris consists of pupillary and ciliary zones. It is supplied by the anterior ciliary arteries, and innervated by branches of the long and short ciliary nerves which are derived from the nasociliary nerve. The iris contains the dilator pupillae and sphincter pupillae, and the former is innervated by non-myelinated sympathetic nerves.[1]
**Difficulty level: 3**

**71**   i. F      ii. T      iii. F      iv. F      v. T

Descemet's layer of the cornea is a thin layer measuring approximately 8–12 μm in thickness. It serves as the layer in between the endothelium and the corneal stroma. The corneal stroma contains thick, flattened collagenous lamellae orientated parallel to the corneal surface. The collagen fibres in the stroma are mainly collagen type 1 although there are some collagen types 3, 5 and 6 present. Bowman's layer supports the corneal epithelium, and this is an acellular region of 8–12 μm thickness. The corneal epithelium itself has no immunocompetent cells and the area is avascular. This is of course vital in relevance to corneal grafting.[1]
**Difficulty level: 3**

**72**   i. F      ii. T      iii. F      iv. T      v. T

In the adult eye the lens typically has an axial length of 4 mm, with a diameter of approximately 10 mm. It becomes rounder with age. The lens capsule is elastic and completely envelops the lens. It consists of basement membrane glycoproteins and glycosaminoglycans (GAGs). The lens epithelium is typically simple cuboidal epithelium, although the cells become more columnar at the equator. Cells in the lens are linked by 'ball and socket' cytoplasmic interdigitations and gap junctions. Lens fibres are rich in cytoskeletal elements, ribosomes and rough endoplasmic reticulum. It is thought that biochemical dysregulation may be one mechanism whereby the natural lens becomes cataractous.[1]
**Difficulty level: 3**

**73**   i.  F      ii.  F      iii.  T      iv.  F      v.  T

The vitreous is a viscoelastic gel, four times the density of water, and consists mainly of water (98%). It is adherent to the pars plana (via the vitreous base), the optic disc and also along major blood vessels. The anterior depression of the vitreous is known as the hyaloid fossa. The vitreous base is a tight 3- to 4-mm band, and the ligamentum hyaloide capsulare attaches to the posterior capsule. The vitreous is divided into two parts – the cortical vitreous is characterised by densely arranged collagen fibres and a central vitreous cavity that is more liquid.[1]
   **Difficulty level: 3**

**74**   i.  T      ii.  T      iii.  F      iv.  T      v.  F

The ciliary body is a ring of tissue that is bordered by the scleral spur and the ora serrata. The ora serrata contains non-pigmented ciliary epithelium. Seen in cross section, the base of the ciliary body faces the anterior chamber and the apex fuses with the choroid. The ciliary body consists of a pars plana and pars plicata – the pars plicata is 2 mm wide and the pars plana is 4 mm wide. The pars plicata consists of many ciliary processes. The ciliary muscle has both longitudinal and meridional elements. The longitudinal muscle is attached to the scleral spur. The fibres are separated when a traumatic cyclodialysis cleft is formed.[1]
   **Difficulty level: 4**

**75**   i.  F      ii.  T      iii.  T      iii.  T      v.  F

The blood supply of the ciliary body occurs from the long posterior ciliary arteries. These are derived from the ophthalmic artery, and traverse forwards through the choroid before anastomosing with the anterior ciliary arteries. The parasympathetic preganglionic nerve cell bodies are situated in the Edinger-Westphal nucleus, eventually synapsing with postganglionic nerve fibres in the ciliary ganglion. Sympathetic innervations are via preganglionic nerves whose cells are located in the lateral grey horn of the first thoracic segment at the level of T1. These fibres then synapse with the superior cervical ganglion, which is typically located at the level of C2 and C3.[1]
   **Difficulty level: 4**

**76**   i. T      ii. T      iii. F      iv. F      v. T

The internal carotid artery has a number of branches, including the ophthalmic artery, the vidian artery (artery of the pterygoid canal), the inferior hypophyseal artery and middle cerebral artery. The vidian artery arises from the cervical part of the internal carotid artery and serves as an anastomosis between it and the external carotid artery. The inferior hypophyseal artery arises from the meningohypophyseal trunk at the level of C4. The middle cerebral artery arises from the communicating section of the internal carotid artery at the level of C7. It goes on to supply many areas of the cerebral cortex, including the temporal lobes.[2]

**Difficulty level: 4**


**77**   i. T      ii. T      iii. T      iv. F      v. T

The superior rectus lies beneath the levator palpebrae superioris and is innervated by the 3rd (oculomotor) cranial nerve. The superior rectus originates from a common tendinous ring along with the medial, inferior and lateral recti. It inserts approximately 7.8 mm from the limbus, the furthest posteriorly of the recti muscles. The length of the muscle tendon is approximately 5.4 mm and the length of the muscle belly approximately 41 mm. The medial rectus inserts most proximally to the limbus at approximately 5.5 mm. The shortest muscle is the superior oblique and longest tendon length is of the lateral rectus (approximately 8.4 mm).[1]

**Difficulty level: 4**


**78**   i. T      ii. F      iii. F      iv. T      v. T

The facial (7th) cranial nerve arises from the second pharyngeal arch and supplies the muscles of facial expression. In addition to this it supplies the stapedius of the middle ear and the anterior two thirds of the tongue. The extracranial branch of the nerve exits the skull through the stylomastoid foramen. It passes through the parotid gland, which is why in cases of trauma and infection of the gland, a facial nerve palsy can result. Another section of the facial nerve is the nervus intermedius, which supplies the lacrimal gland.[1]

**Difficulty level: 4**

**79**   i.  T      ii.  F      iii.  T      iv.  F      v.  T

The occipitofrontalis muscle consists of two occipital bellies posteriorly attached through a thick fibrous layer to the anterior bellies via the galea aponeurotica. The anterior section inserts into the superficial fascia of the eyelids. The frontal section is supplied, like other muscles of facial expression, by the facial nerve. The depressor supercilii are fibres of the orbicularis oculi that are inserted into the skin and connective tissue of the eyebrow. The levator palpebrae superioris is innervated by the oculomotor cranial nerve and originates from the lesser wing of sphenoid. It also fuses with the origin of the superior rectus.[1]
   **Difficulty level: 4**

**80**   i.  T      ii.  T      iii.  T      iv.  F      v.  T

The lacrimal gland lies superotemporal to the globe and consists of two sections, a larger orbital section and smaller, palpebral portion. It is supplied by the lacrimal artery and branches of the infraorbital artery derived from the external carotid artery. Venous drainage is usually via ophthalmic veins rather than the vortex veins. Lymph drainage from the lacrimal gland occurs to the preauricular lymph node. The lacrimal gland is innervated by descending autonomic pathways that control tear production. Reflex watering is initiated by the irritation of the cornea, and interneurones connect the trigeminal sensory nuclei with the lacrimatory nucleus.[1]
   **Difficulty level: 3**

**81**   i.  T      ii.  F      iii.  T      iv.  T      v.  F

The optic nerve is supplied by the ophthalmic artery and some branches of the hypophyseal artery. The optic chiasm is supplied by the superior hypophyseal and branches from the internal carotid artery. The lateral root of the optic tract is supplied by the anterior choroidal artery. The lateral geniculate nucleus is supplied by the anterior choroidal artery as well as branches of the posterior cerebral artery. The optic radiation is supplied by the anterior choroidal artery. The visual cortex is supplied by branches of the posterior cerebral artery, and perforating branches of the cortical arteries.[1]
   **Difficulty level: 4**

**82**   i. T     ii. F     iii. T     iv. F     v. T

Lymphatic drainage of the eyelid is to the superficial parotid or submandibular lymph nodes. The arterial supply to the eyelid is derived by two arteries – the pretarsal eyelid is supplied by the superficial temporal and facial arteries, and the post-tarsal eyelid is supplied by the ophthalmic artery. Venous drainage of the eyelid is via the ophthalmic veins, and these go on to drain into the cavernous sinus.[1]

**Difficulty level: 3**

**83**   i. F     ii. T     iii. T     iv. F     v. F

The ophthalmic artery is derived from the internal carotid artery and has numerous branches within the orbit. The artery eventually terminates as the dorsal nasal artery and trochlear arteries. Posterior ciliary arteries are derived from the ophthalmic artery and divide into four long posterior ciliary arteries and up to seven or more short posterior ciliary arteries. The lacrimal artery is a branch of the ophthalmic artery. The veins of the orbit are devoid of valves and this is of importance, clinically, in terms of the spread of infection. The inferior ophthalmic vein drains to the pterygoid venous plexus.[1]

**Difficulty level: 4**

**84**   i. T     ii. F     iii. F     iv. T     v. T

The primary visual cortex is situated either side of the calcarine sulcus. The macula projects posteriorly and the peripheral retina anteriorly. Input is primarily from the ipsilateral lateral geniculate nucleus. Only cells after the first synapse in the primary visual cortex receive binocular input. Like the cerebral cortex elsewhere, the primary visual cortex has six layers. Layer V projects to the superior colliculus.[3]

**Difficulty level: 3**

**85**   i. T     ii. F     iii. T     iv. T     v. T

Saccades are the fastest of eye movements and have a velocity of up to 400 degrees per second. Horizontal saccades are controlled by the frontal eye fields in area 8 of the frontal cortex, from where impulses pass to the parapontine reticular formation, the start of the final common pathway of horizontal eye movements, and onto the various oculomotor nuclei. The vertical gaze centre is less well understood but thought to lie in the rostral interstitial nucleus of the medial longitudinal fasciculus.[4]

**Difficulty level: 4**

**86**    i. T      ii. T      iii. F      iv. F      v. T

The trochlear nerve has the longest intracranial course of any cranial nerve at approximately 75 mm. The trochlear nerve passes forwards in the lateral wall of the cavernous sinus. It enters the orbit through the superior orbital fissure outside the annulus of Zinn.[5]

**Difficulty level: 2**

**87**    i. F      ii. T      iii. T      iv. T      v. F

The abducens cranial nerve is a motor nerve. In the cavernous sinus, it may transiently carry sympathetic fibres from the carotid plexus. The abducens nerve supplies the lateral rectus.[5]

**Difficulty level: 2**

**88**    i. T      ii. T      iii. T      iv. F      v. T

Lymphatic vessels drain the eyelids to the preauricular and submandibular nodes. No orbital lymphatic vessels have been demonstrated, although orbital oedema may resolve.[6]

**Difficulty level: 3**

**89**    i. F      ii. F      iii. T      iv. T      v. T

The internal capsule runs laterally to the LGN. The LGN consists of six layers of grey matter. Layers 1 and 2 contribute to the magnocellular pathway and layers 3 to 6 the parvocellular pathway.[4]

**Difficulty level: 3**

**90**    i. T      ii. F      iii. F      iv. T      v. T

The facial nerve supplies the muscles of facial expression. It provides sensation to the anterior two-thirds of the tongue and the external auditory canal. It also provides parasympathetic innervations for the lacrimal gland and salivation.

The muscles of mastication are supplied by the motor component of the trigeminal nerve.[5]
   **Difficulty level: 2**


**91**   i.  F      ii.  F      iii.  F      iv.  T      v.  T

Lesions posterior to the chiasm cause homonymous field defects as nerve fibres from the two eyes have crossed.[3]
   **Difficulty level: 2**


**92**   i.  T      ii.  F      iii.  F      iv.  T      v.  F

Parasympathetic fibres in the short ciliary nerves are postganglionic. Sympathetic vasomotor fibres also pass to the eye via the short ciliary nerves. Sympathetic fibres originate in the hypothalamus and medulla.[3]
   **Difficulty level: 5**


**93**   i.  T      ii.  F      iii.  T      iv.  F      v.  T

The spinal nerve carries pain and temperature. The lacrimal branch of the trigeminal nerve lies at the upper border of the lateral rectus muscle.[5]
   **Difficulty level: 4**


**94**   i.  T      ii.  F      iii.  F      iv.  T      v.  T

The superior salivatory nucleus supplies fibres to the lacrimal gland, submandibular gland, sublingual gland, nasal mucosa and pharynx. The inferior salivatory nucleus supplies fibres to the parotid gland.[5]
   **Difficulty level: 4**


**95**   i.  T      ii.  F      iv.  F      iv.  T      v.  T

The optic chiasm lies inferior to the floor of the third ventricle. The chiasm is superior to the diaphragma sellae. The chiasm has the cavernous sinus and internal carotid artery lateral to it.[3]
   **Difficulty level: 3**

**96**  i. F      ii. T      iii. T      iv. F      v. T

The left common carotid artery arises from the aortic arch. The right common carotid artery arises from the brachiocephalic artery. The external carotid artery enters the parotid gland. The superficial temporal artery and maxillary artery are terminal branches of the external carotid artery.[7]
  **Difficulty level: 3**

**97**  i. T      ii. T      iii. T      iv. F      v. T

The temporal crescent of the visual field is monocular and therefore has no dominance columns. Monocular deprivation in early life leads to uneven distribution of dominance columns.[8]
  **Difficulty level: 4**

**98**  i. T      ii. T      iii. F      iv. T      v. T

There is no direct projection from the visual cortex to the retina. Areas 18 and 19 represent the secondary visual area. Wernicke's area receives fibres from the visual cortex of the occipital lobe and the auditory cortex in the superior temporal gyrus, permitting understanding of written and spoken language.[6]
  **Difficulty level: 4**

**99**  i. T      ii. F      iii. F      iv. T      v. F

Accommodation is characterised by the triad of convergence, pupil constriction and thickening of the lens (increasing its refractive power) by contraction of the ciliary muscle. Parasympathetic fibres are involved in the efferent pathway of the accommodative reflex, beginning in the Edinger-Westphal nucleus, synapsing in the ciliary ganglion, with postganglionic fibres passing in the short ciliary nerve to the ciliary muscles and sphincter pupillae.[6]
  **Difficulty level: 3**

**100**  i. F      ii. F      iii. T      iv. T      v. T

The orbital venous system is independent of the arterial system. The orbital venous system is devoid of valves. There are three major outflow pathways – the cavernous sinus, pterygoid plexus and anterior venous system with connections to the angular vein.[6]
  **Difficulty level: 4**

# References

1 Forrester J, Dick A, McMenamin A, *et al. The Eye: basic sciences in practice*. 2nd ed. Philadelphia: Saunders Elsevier; 2007. (**q51**) p. 5, (**q52**) pp. 7–8, (**q53**) pp. 64–5, (**q54**) p. 60, (**q55**) pp. 84–6, (**q56**) pp. 88–90, (**q57**) pp. 18–19, (**q58**) pp. 35–8, (**q59**) pp. 66–7, (**q60**) pp. 48–50, (**q61**) pp. 45–6, (**q62**) pp. 40–1, (**q63**) pp. 23–6, (**q64**) pp. 42–3, (**q65**) pp. 67–9, (**q66**) pp. 75–7, (**q67**) pp. 77–9, (**q68**) pp. 2–4, (**q69**) pp. 10–11, (**q70**) pp. 26–7, (**q71**) pp. 17–20, (**q72**) pp. 30–3, (**q73**) pp. 36–7, (**q74**) pp. 30–2, (**q75**) pp. 30–1, (**q77**) p. 65, (**q78**) pp. 76–7, (**q79**) pp. 78–9, (**q80**) pp. 86–7, (**q81**) pp. 92–3, (**q82**) pp. 80–1, (**q83**) pp. 66–7.

2 Bouthillier A, Van Loveren H, Jefferey K. Segments of the internal carotid artery: a new classification. *Neurosurgery*. 1996; **38**(3): 425–32 (**q76**).

3 Crossman A, Neary D. *Neuroanatomy – an illustrated colour text*. 2nd ed. Philadelphia: Churchill Livingstone; 2000. (**q84**) p. 164, (**q91**) p. 165, (**q92**) p. 106, (**q95**) p. 163.

4 Kline L. *Neuro-Ophthalmology Review Manual*. 6th ed. New Jersey: Slack; 2008. (**q85**) p. 47, (**q89**) p. 5.

5 Weiss J. *Fundamentals and Principles of Ophthalmology. Part III: Cranial nerves*. San Francisco: American Academy of Ophthalmology Basic and Clinical Science Course 2010–11. (**q86**) p. 106, (**q87, q93**), p. 104, (**q90**) p. 105, (**q94**) p. 108.

6 Snell R, Lemp M. *Clinical Anatomy of the Eye*. 2nd ed. Malden: Blackwell Publishing; 2006. (**q88**) p. 102, (**q98**) p. 398, (**q99**) p. 370, (**q100**) pp. 287–8.

7 Moore K, Dalley A. *Clinically Orientated Anatomy*. 4th ed. Philadelphia: Lippincott, Williams & Wilkins; 1999. (**q96**) pp. 1017–18.

8 Purves D, Augustine G, Fitzpatrick D. *Neuroscience*. 2nd ed. Sunderland, MA: Sinauer; 2001. (**q97**) p. 525.

# 2. Physiology FRCOphth answers

1 **A** For an 'average' 70-kg man, the volume of plasma water is approximately 3 L, interstitial water is 11 L, total extracellular volume (i.e. plasma and interstitial) is 14 L and intracellular water is 28 L.[1]
**Difficulty level: 2**

2 **D** The concentration of potassium in extracellular fluid is 4 mmol/L, and 140 mmol/L in intracellular fluid. That of sodium is 14 mmol/L in intracellular fluid and 142 mmol/L in extracellular fluid.[1]
**Difficulty level: 2**

3 **B** The resting potential of a nerve fibre is the voltage difference across the plasma membrane and is approximately –90 mV. The distribution of all ions across the membrane contributes; however, potassium ions have the greatest effect since potassium has the highest permeability across the cell membrane.[1]
**Difficulty level: 2**

4 **D** Depolarisation of nerve cells following an action potential causes opening of voltage-gated calcium channels. Calcium plays an important role in the mobilisation of vesicles containing neurotransmitter and fusion with the presynaptic membrane.[1]
**Difficulty level: 3**

5 **B** Eosinophils are involved in combating parasitic infection, and in the mechanisms associated with allergy.[2]
**Difficulty level: 2**

6 **C** Protein C is a normal component of the clotting cascade and activates Va and VIIIa. Protein C deficiency promotes thrombosis. Lupus anticoagulant prolongs activated partial thromboplastin time (APTT) in vitro but is prothrombotic in vivo. Factor V Leiden and homocysteinaemia are also prothrombotic.[2]
**Difficulty level: 3**

7 **D** Autoregulatory mechanisms maintain a constant blood flow to organs. Reduction in oxygen concentration, reduction in pH and increase in carbon dioxide concentration cause vasodilation and increased blood flow (with the exception of the pulmonary vasculature where the opposite occurs). Raised blood pressure causes reflex vasoconstriction to regulate blood flow.[1]
**Difficulty level: 3**

8 **A** Blood pressure = cardiac output × total peripheral resistance
Cardiac output = stroke volume × heart rate
Stroke volume = end diastolic volume – end systolic volume
Therefore, A is the correct answer as increased end systolic volume results in decreased stroke volume, so reduced cardiac output and therefore blood pressure.[1,3]
**Difficulty level: 4**

9 **B** Vital capacity is the maximum volume of air that can be respired. It is the difference between total lung capacity and reserve volume; or the total sum of tidal volume, inspiratory and expiratory reserve volume.[1]
**Difficulty level: 3**

10 **C** Oxygen is transported in combination with haemoglobin in the blood and oxyhaemoglobin has a sigmoidal dissociation curve. High temperature, acidosis and increased $pCO_2$ cause the dissociation curve to shift to the right, thereby encouraging oxygen to be offloaded to the tissue. Carbon monoxide has a higher affinity for haemoglobin than oxygen and so causes a shift to the left.[1]
**Difficulty level: 3**

11 **B** The pituitary synthesises prolactin, growth hormone, ACTH, luteinising hormone, follicle-stimulating hormone and thyroid-stimulating hormone. Oxytocin and antidiuretic hormone are synthesised in the hypothalamus and then transported down nerve axons to be released by the posterior pituitary. Growth hormone-releasing hormone is produced by the hypothalamus.[1]
**Difficulty level: 3**

12 **B** Insulin promotes glycogen synthesis (whereas glucagon promotes glycogen breakdown) in the liver. It also promotes lipogenesis and inhibits lipolysis. Insulin is produced by the beta cells in the islets of Langerhans.[1]
**Difficulty level: 2**

13 **D** Vitamin A deficiency may cause night blindness, xerophthalmia (severe dry eye leading to corneal keratinisation) and keratomalacia. Vitamin $B_1$ deficiency is associated with Wernicke's encephalopathy, features of which are nystagmus and ophthalmoplegia. Vitamin $B_{12}$ is associated with optic atrophy, especially in alcoholics. Vitamin K deficiency prolongs bleeding time – warfarin works by interfering with the action of vitamin K.[3]
**Difficulty level: 4**

14 **A** Aldosterone acts to restore circulating volume. Therefore, it causes sodium reabsorption (leading to retention of water) and potassium excretion (thus hypokalaemia if secreted in excess). It acts on the distal tubule of the nephron.[1]
**Difficulty level: 3**

15 **C** Acetylcholine is the only neurotransmitter in autonomic ganglia.[1]
**Difficulty level: 4**

**16 B**  Pepsin is released, by chief cells of the stomach, in its inactive pro-enzyme form pepsinogen. It is activated to pepsin by the high hydrogen ion concentration in the gastric lumen.[1]
**Difficulty level: 3**

**17 C**  The physiological range for serum platelets is 150–400 × 10⁹/L. The lifespan of circulating platelets is 5–9 days. Platelets are derived from megakaryocytes, and are regulated by thrombospondin.[1]
**Difficulty level: 3**

**18 A**  Melatonin is produced by the pineal gland in the brain, and permits circadian sleep-wake cycles. Current research is being focused upon its use in the treatment of delirium and attention deficit hypersensitivity disorder.[6]
**Difficulty level: 3**

**19 C**  Corneal transparency is a function of the relative acellularity and matrix structure of the stroma. Collagen type I, the most predominant type of collagen in the stroma, is regularly arranged and this is also considered important in transparency.[4]
**Difficulty level: 3**

**20 A**  Glucose enters lens cells via an insulin-dependent glucose transporter. About 80% of glucose is consumed by the lens via anaerobic glycolysis. In an environment where glucose is in high concentrations, the sorbitol pathway is used.[4]
**Difficulty level: 3**

**21 C**  The rate of aqueous humour formation is 2–3 uL/min. Aqueous humour is formed by water and electrolytes from leaky capillaries of the ciliary processes. This fluid then passes through the plasma membrane of the non-pigmented epithelium.[4]
**Difficulty level: 2**

**22 C**  The Imbert-Fick principle states that the pressure inside an idealised sphere is equal to the force required to flatten the surface divided by the area of flattening.[5]
**Difficulty level: 2**

**23 A**  The major glycosaminoglycan is keratan sulphate, whilst smaller amounts of chondroitin sulphate and non-sulphated chondroitin are also present.[4]
**Difficulty level: 4**

**24 C** The refractive index of the vitreous is in fact 1.33. It consists of predominantly water (98%), 1.0% macromolecules and the remainder consists of solutes and low molecular weight materials.[4]
**Difficulty level: 3**

**25 D** Zona occludens attach RPE cells to each other to form the blood-retinal barrier. This barrier makes the retina impermeable to the passage of molecules larger than 30 000 Da.[4]
**Difficulty level: 3**

**26 A** Activation of rhodospin occurs via the isomerisation of retinol, which is a Vitamin A compound. Eleven-cis (11-cis) retinal becomes converted to all-trans-retinal in the first steps of phototransduction.[4]
**Difficulty level: 4**

**27 C** Glucagon is thought to act as a neuromodulator within amacrine cells. Glutamate is the major neurotransmitter, taurine acts upon horizontal amacrine cells, and thyrotropin-releasing hormone acts upon amacrine and ganglion cells.[4]
**Difficulty level: 5**

**28 A** Dopamine is present in amacrine cells, and exerts a neuromodulatory effect on retinal function. However, dopamine receptors are present on a variety of retinal neurones and so dopamine may have a number of unidentified functions, yet to be discovered. Dopamine may be responsible for the regulation of spatial contrast sensitivity in view of its presence in amacrine cells.[4]
**Difficulty level: 3**

**29 A** Alpha-2 ($\alpha$-2) selective adrenergic agonists suppress aqueous flow via an inhibition of adenylate cyclase, and act on $\alpha$-2 receptors which are located in the ciliary body. By stimulating $\beta$ receptors there is an increase in aqueous secretion through the stimulation of adenylate cyclase.[4]
**Difficulty level: 4**

**30 A** Luminosity and hue are not independent, and as the luminosity of the stimulus increases all hues appear yellow-white. This is known as the Bezold-Brücke phenomenon. All hues appear achromatic as the intensity of the light decreases. This is known as the Purkinje shift.[4]
**Difficulty level: 5**

**31 B** A horopter is essential for binocular single vision, and can be mapped by the corresponding single points joined together. The vertical horopter

has a backward tilt that passes through the point of fixation and a point near the feet of the observer. Panum's area is the range of angular disparities where the vision is single and fused – it encompasses a larger area horizontally compared to vertically and so forms an ellipse.[4]
**Difficulty level: 4**

32  **A**   The oculomotor cerebellar centre is located in lobules VI and VII of the cerebellum, and input is derived from the pontine paramedian reticular formation (PPRF). Purkinje cells are important for the initiation of saccadic-type movements.[4]
**Difficulty level: 4**

33  **C**   It is hypothesised that cortical blindness may also be due to problems with visual processing. Cortical lesions in the superior temporal sulcus can affect motion perception. Similarly, lesions to the lingual or fusiform gyrus are associated with prosopagnosia (an inability to recognise faces).[4]
**Difficulty level: 5**

34  **D**   The eye acts as a dipole and the resting potential can be measured between the retinal pigment epithelium and photoreceptors. In a light adapted state the potential rises. This resting potential is lost when the adhesion between the retinal pigment epithelium and the photoreceptors is disrupted.[4]
**Difficulty level: 4**

35  **C**   Colour discrimination varies across the spectrum and across the visual field according to the frequency distribution of the three cones. Colour discrimination is maximal at the fovea and mid-spectrum. The rods are not involved in colour vision.[4]
**Difficulty level: 4**

36  **C**   The genes for green (medium wavelength) and red (long wavelength) pigment are found on the X chromosome. Therefore, 8% of males have congenital colour vision defects, largely because of X-linked recessive disease. The gene for blue (short wavelength) pigment is found on chromosome 7 and therefore congenital colour defects affecting blue pigment are rarer.[7]
**Difficulty level: 4**

37  **C**   The angle of image disparity gives rise to binocular parallax contributing to binocular depth perception.[4]
**Difficulty level: 4**

**38 D** Approximately 80% of ganglion cell axons pass in the parvocellular pathway and 10% in the magnocellular pathway.[4]
**Difficulty level: 4**

**39 A** The role of saccades is to bring an object of interest to the fovea. Saccades are under supranuclear contralateral control. Saccades can be voluntary or reflex. Latency is long – over 100 ms. Velocity can be rapid, around 800 degrees per second – the fastest of all eye movements.[4]
**Difficulty level: 3**

**40 D** The role of smooth pursuit movements is to hold the image to the fovea. These tracking movements start to break down with targets moving at a velocity greater than 40 degrees per second. Smooth pursuit is stimulated by movement of the target image across the foveal and parafoveal retina (retinal slip).[4]
**Difficulty level: 4**

**41 B** Vernier hyperacuity describes the phenomenon of being able to detect a break in a line subtending less than 10 seconds of arc. Even though the minimum cone separation in the macula is 1 minute of arc, cortical processing allows this fine degree of discrimination.[4]
**Difficulty level: 3**

**42 D** The physiological blind spot is about 10–20 degrees temporal to the centre of the visual field. It corresponds to the area of the optic nerve head where photoreceptors are absent.[8]
**Difficulty level: 1**

**43 C** Adie's tonic pupil is most common in young adults. It has a female predilection. Eighty per cent are present unilaterally initially, with it tending to become bilateral at a rate of 4% per year.[8]
**Difficulty level: 2**

**44 C** Remember the mnemonic 'COWS' – cold-opposite and warm-same side in reference to the fast phase of nystagmus on caloric testing.[8]
**Difficulty level: 2**

**45 B** Supranuclear control of vertical saccades originates in the frontal eye fields or superior colliculus. They project to the nuclei of cranial nerves III and IV via the rostral interstitial nucleus of the medial longitudinal fasciculus (MLF). The paramedian pontine reticular formation (PPRF) controls horizontal eye movements.[8]
**Difficulty level: 4**

**46 B** Uhthoff's phenomenon occurs with optic neuritis and may be triggered by exercise or hot showers. It is suspected that the increase in temperature slows nerve conduction and that with demyelination this effect is amplified. Lhermitte's sign is an electric shock sensation noted on neck flexion and associated with multiple sclerosis.[9]
**Difficulty level: 3**

**47 D** The pattern ERG is derived from the central retina and the $P_{50}$ component is invariably affected in macula disease. In contrast, optic nerve disease will only affect the $N_{95}$ component if there has been significant retrograde degeneration to the retinal ganglion cells.[5]
**Difficulty level: 4**

**48 A** One dilated pupil does not prevent detection of a relative afferent pupillary defect. Because the pupillary efferents are equal bilaterally, the consensual light response can be used instead of the direct response to detect an afferent defect. A relative afferent pupillary defect does not directly cause anisocoria because the pupillary fibres decussate in the chiasm and posterior commissure to ensure equal efferent input to both iris sphincter muscles.[5]
**Difficulty level: 2**

**49 B** The different temporal and light sensitivities of the rod and cone systems can be used to isolate their particular contributions to the ERG. A bright background can be used to saturate the rod system and give a cone-only response. Only the cone system can respond to stimuli at frequencies greater than 20 Hz. The ERG response to a single flash of white light is a combined rod-and-cone response.[5]
**Difficulty level: 3**

**50 C** In an amblyopic eye, the flash VEP will usually be normal (as a focused image is not required), whereas the pattern VEP (reversing chequerboard pattern) will usually be abnormal. The flash VEP can be used in patient groups with low cooperation, such as young children. As the stimulus is presented monocularly and responses over both occipital cortices are measured, this allows the degree of crossover at the chiasm to be assessed. In albinism, for example, there is increased crossover at the chiasm.[5]
**Difficulty level: 4**

## References

1 Guyton AC, Hall J. *Textbook of Medical Physiology*. 11th ed. Philadelphia: Saunders Elsevier; 2006. (**q1**) p. 292, (**q2**) p. 294, (**q3**) pp. 59–61, (**q4**) p. 560, (**q7**) pp. 219–20, (**q8**) p. 234, (**q9**) pp. 475–6, (**q10**) pp. 506–8, (**q11**) pp. 919–21, (**q12**) pp. 964–5, (**q14**) pp. 948–9, (**q15**) p. 750, (**q16**) pp. 797–800, (**q17**) pp. 425–30.

2 Kumar P, Abbas A, Fausto N, *et al. Robbins and Cotran Pathologic Basis of Disease*. 8th ed. Philadelphia: Saunders Elsevier; 2010, (**q5**) p. 75, (**q6**) p. 122.

3 Colledge NR, Walker BR, Ralston SH. *Davidson's Principles and Practice of Medicine*. 21st ed. Edinburgh: Churchill Livingstone Elsevier; 2010. (**q8**) p. 527, (**q13**) pp. 125–8.

4 Forrester J, Dick A, McMenamin A, *et al. The Eye: basic sciences in practice*. 2nd ed. Philadelphia: Saunders Elsevier; 2007. (**q19**) pp. 178–80, (**q20**) pp. 200–1, (**q21**) pp. 192–3, (**q23**) pp. 178–81, (**q24**) pp. 204–6, (**q25**) pp. 208–13, (**q26**) pp. 216–18, (**q27, q28**) pp. 220–2, (**q29**) pp. 194–5, (**q30**) pp. 224–6, (**q31**) pp. 248–9, (**q32**) pp. 262–3, (**q33**) pp. 244–5, (**q34**) pp. 238–9, (**q35**) pp. 252–4, (**q37**) p. 248, (**q38**) p. 254, (**q39**) pp. 256–60, (**q40**) p. 258, (**q41**) p. 229.

5 Madge S, Kersey J, Hawker M, *et al. Clinical Techniques in Ophthalmology*. Edinburgh: Churchill Livingstone; 2006. (**q22**) pp. 132–5, (**q47**) p. 161, (**q48**) pp. 111–12, (**q49**) p. 160, (**q50**) p. 163.

6 Al-Aama T, Brymer C, Gutmanis I, *et al*. Melatonin decreases delirium in elderly patients: a randomized, placebo-controlled trial. *Intl J Geriatr Psychiatry*. 2011; **26**(7): 687–94 (**q18**).

7 Purves D, Augustine G, Fitzpatrick D, *et al. Neuroscience*. 2nd ed. Sunderland, MA: Sinauer; 2000. (**q36**) p. 241.

8 Kline LB, *Neuro-Ophthalmology Review Manual*. 6th ed. New Jersey: Slack; 2007. (**q42**) p. 1, (**q43**) p. 131, (**q44**) p. 61, (**q45**) p. 50.

9 White LJ, Dressendorfer LH. Exercise and multiple sclerosis. *Sports Med*. 2004; **34**(15): 1077–100 (**q46**).

# 2. Physiology ICO answers

**51**   i. T      ii. F      iii. F      iv. T      v. T

Vitamin A is present as a provitamin in the yellow and red carotenoid pigments in vegetables such as carrots. It is fat soluble and so deficiency may occur in malabsorption syndromes. The provitamin is converted into retinol in the liver and stores in the liver may last for 5 to 10 months. Vitamin A deficiency is the leading cause of childhood blindness worldwide. Features include night blindness, xerosis (drying) of the conjunctiva and then cornea due to loss of goblet cells, and eventually corneal ulceration and perforation. Treatment is with high-dose vitamin A.[1,2]

**Difficulty level: 3**

**52**   i. F        ii. T        iii. F        iv. T        v. T

The original age-related eye disease study (AREDS) established the combination of zinc, beta-carotene and vitamins C and E in reducing the progression of age-related macular degeneration. Subsequently lutein, zeaxanthin, B vitamins, and omega-3 fatty acids have also been associated with reduced progression. The AREDS 2 study is currently underway.[3]

**Difficulty level: 4**

**53**   i. F        ii. T        iii. F        iv. F        v. T

In hyperthyroidism there is elevated free $T_4$ and due to negative feedback, TSH is subsequently suppressed. In hypothyroidism there is low free $T_4$ and elevated TSH. Positive thyroid-peroxidase antibodies are associated with Graves' disease and also Hashimoto's thyroiditis.[4]

**Difficulty level: 3**

**54**   i. F        ii. T        iii. F        iv. F        v. T

Osmotic pressure is the hydrostatic pressure required to oppose the movement of water through a semipermeable membrane in response to an osmotic gradient. Oncotic pressure or colloidal osmotic pressure is the component of osmotic pressure exerted by large molecular weight particles such as proteins in plasma. Albumin contributes 80%, globulin around 20% and a very small amount from fibrinogen. The oncotic pressure of plasma is around 28 mmHg.[2]

**Difficulty level: 3**

**55**   i. T        ii. F        iii. F        iv. T        v. T

The sarcolemma is the cell membrane of the muscle fibre. Each muscle fibre contains several hundred to a thousand myofibrils which consist of thick myosin filaments and thin actin filaments. These interdigitate and are responsible for muscle contraction. Actin filaments are attached to the Z disc and extend from both sides of the Z disc to interact with myosin filaments. The areas where only actin is present are called I bands as they are isotropic to polarised light. The areas where myosin is present are called A bands. The distance between two Z discs defines the sarcomere.[2]

**Difficulty level: 4**

**56**    i. T       ii. F       iii. F       iv. F       v. T

When the action potential travelling down the motor nerve reaches its terminal, acteylcholine (ACh) is released. ACh passes across the synapse and binds to nicotinic ACh receptors on the motor end plate. There is sodium influx into the muscle fibre via these channels, which initiates an action potential. This depolarises the muscle fibre, which causes calcium release from the sarcoplasmic reticulum. Calcium binds to troponin C on the actin filaments and initiates sliding of the actin and myosin filaments and thus contraction.[2]

**Difficulty level: 3**

**57**    i. F       ii. T       iii. T       iv. T       v. T

Haemolytic anaemia may be congenital or acquired. Congenital causes include hereditary spherocytosis, sickle-cell anaemia, thalassaemia and glucose-6-phosphate deficiency. Acquired causes include immune, mechanical (such as artificial heart valves), malaria and drugs.[5]

**Difficulty level: 3**

**58**    i. F       ii. F       iii. F       iv. F       v. F

The rate of flow in a blood vessel is described by Poiseuille's law:

$$\text{Rate of blood flow} = \frac{\varpi \Delta P r4}{8 \eta l}$$

Where $\Delta P$ is the difference in pressure between the two ends of the vessel, r is radius, $\eta$ is viscosity and l is vessel length. Therefore, larger vessel diameter, larger pressure difference, shorter vessel length and lower viscosity increase blood flow.[2]

**Difficulty level: 3**

**59**  i. F    ii. T    iii. F    iv. T    v. F

The presynaptic membrane contains voltage-gated calcium channels. Calcium binds to release sites in the presynaptic terminal leading to exocytosis of synaptic vesicles containing neurotransmitter. Examples of neurotransmitters include acetylcholine, adrenaline, noradrenaline, GABA and glutamate. Postsynaptic receptors may be ion channels or G-protein coupled receptors. Sodium influx into the postsynaptic cell is excitatory; potassium and chloride influx into the post-synaptic cell are inhibitory.[2]

**Difficulty level: 3**

**60**  i. T    ii. F    iii. T    iv. F    v. T

Pain receptors are free nerve endings. Mechanical, chemical and thermal stimuli are able to activate pain receptors. Bradykinin, serotonin, histamine and acetylcholine, amongst other mediators, activate chemical pain receptors. Prostaglandins and substance P enhance sensitivity of pain receptors but do not directly excite them. Pain receptors show little adaptation and in some cases repeated excitation leads to increased sensitivity, which is seen as hyperalgesia.[2]

**Difficulty level: 3**

**61**  i. T    ii. F    iii. T    iv. T    v. T

Basal secretion of tears occurs via a sodium/potassium ATPase pump, a sodium/potassium/chloride co-transporter, potassium channels in the basal membrane of the acinar cell and chloride channels in the apical membrane. The rate of basal tear secretion is 1.2 μL/min.

Stimulated tear secretion occurs via the autonomic nervous system, with parasympathetic stimulation increasing tear production. Acetylcholine release stimulates muscarinic acetylcholine receptors to mobilise calcium stores, resulting in the opening of potassium and chloride channels. The accessory lacrimal glands constantly produce tears. Conjunctival sac volume is 25–30 μL.[6,7]

**Difficulty level: 4**

**62**  i. T    ii. T    iii. T    iv. F    v. T

The vitreous contains hyaluronic acid, amino acids, proteins, salts and amino acids. Type 2 collagen forms fine fibrils, which provide a scaffold for the vitreous. The cortex contains more collagen than the central vitreous. With increasing age, the vitreous degenerates and liquefies.[6]

**Difficulty level: 3**


**63**   i. F      ii. F      iii. T      iv. F      v. T

The choroid consists of the vessel layer, capillary layer and Bruch's membrane. It is thickest at the posterior pole. Its main blood supply is from the posterior ciliary arteries, and the main function of the choroid is to supply the outer retina with nutrients. Pigment cells in the choroid absorb excess light that has passed through the retina to prevent reflection of light.[6]

**Difficulty level: 3**


**64**   i. F      ii. T      iii. F      iv. T      v. T

The blood-ocular barrier consists of the blood-aqueous and blood-retinal barriers, which prevent large molecular substances entering the eye. It may be breached by ocular inflammation. The blood-aqueous barrier is formed by tight junctions between non-pigmented ciliary epithelial cells. Tight junctions between non-fenestrated endothelial cells of iris capillaries may also contribute. Regarding the blood-retinal barrier, the outer retina is protected by the tight junctions between retinal pigment epithelial cells. The inner retina is protected by tight junctions between the endothelial cells of capillaries.[6]

**Difficulty level: 3**


**65**   i. T      ii. T      iii. F      iv. F      v. F

Regarding sympathetic stimulation of the heart, noradrenaline is the major transmitter involved. Its release leads to increased sodium and calcium permeability of the muscle fibre membrane. The increased calcium leads to increased force of contraction since calcium plays an important role in cardiac myofibril contraction. The rate of sinus node discharge and the rate of conduction within the heart are increased.[2]

**Difficulty level: 2**


**66**   i. F      ii. T      iii. F      iv. F      v. F

Photoreceptor cells hyperpolarise in the light state following the closure of cGMP-gated sodium ion channels.[7]

**Difficulty level: 4**

**67**   i. T      ii. T      iii. T      iv. T      v. F

Rapid eye movements, fast-phase nystagmus, vestibular nystagmus, refixation nystagmus and optokinetic nystagmus are all examples of saccadic eye movements. Saccadic eye movements are necessary to track objects that are moving at 40 degrees/second or more. Microsaccades are usually associated with refixation and are small 'flicks' of around 4.5 minutes of arc. Imaging studies have suggested that saccadic eye movements probably originate in the contralateral eye fields. Ipsilateral saccades can also be initiated from these areas. On clinical examination, patients with frontocortical cerebral disease often have a deficiency in saccadic function.[8]

**Difficulty level: 5**

**68**   i. T      ii. F      iii. T      iv. F      v. T

Photoreceptor cells are typically bipolar in form and their cell bodies lie in the outer nuclear layer. Synaptic terminals lie at the outer aspect of the outer synaptic/plexiform layer. An elongated section of the cell divides into two portions: the inner segment connects to the cell body within the retina, and the outer segment abuts the inner retinal pigment epithelium. Nine pairs of microtubules lie within the ciliary stalk and this attaches the inner to the outer segments. The apex of the inner segment is a large collection of mitochondria and this area is known as the ellipsoid area. The rest of the ellipsoid area contains ribosomes and Golgi apparatus.[8]

**Difficulty level: 4**

**69**   i. F      ii. T      iii. T      iv. F      v. F

Human tears typically have a pH of 7.4. They contain a number of immuno-globulins and lysozyme enzymes which act in defence of the immediate environment. Lyzozyme makes up 21%–25% of total protein and is decreased in Sjögren's syndrome. The action of lysozyme is heavily dependent on the pH. A total of 12 enzymes have been detected in human tears, including lactate dehydrogenase, amylase and pyruvate kinase. The refractive index of tears is 1.357. Tears contain numerous substances including albumin, globulins and ammonia. Electrolytes that predominate in human tears include bicarbonate, chloride, sodium, potassium and calcium.[8]

**Difficulty level: 4**

**70**   i. T     ii. T     iii. F     iv. F     v. F

The lens is typically dehydrated in vivo, and uses an active pumping mechanism to maintain high concentrations of potassium ions and low levels of sodium ions. Glucose metabolism generates ATP and this is essential for Na/K pumps. Amino acids are actively transported into the lens and are incorporated into the RNA to form lens protein. The turnover of amino acids is rapid. Kynurenine is an amino acid that is thought to play an important role in the absorption of ultraviolet light. Glutathione, a polypeptide, is synthesised within the lens, the vast majority of which is in the deoxidised form. The lipid content of the lens (the majority of which is cholesterol) is variable, representing 3%–5% of the lens.[8]
**Difficulty level: 5**


**71**   i. F     ii. T     iii. T     iv. T     v. F

Many types of amacrine cells have been identified in the human retina. Amacrine II cells release the inhibitory transmitter glycine and these cells also link rod bipolar cells to ganglion cells. Another type of amacrine cells, starburst cells, release acetylcholine at the start and end of a bright stimulus. Dopaminergic cells are postsynaptic to cone bipolar cells and other amacrine cells. Amacrine II cells also make gap junctions with depolarising bipolar cells that contact ganglion cells.

GABA is the most concentrated neurotransmitter in the retina and it is present in both amacrine as well as horizontal cells. Several types of ganglion cell exist, and their density and distribution determines the spatial resolution of the visual system.[7]
**Difficulty level: 5**


**72**   i. T     ii. F     iii. F     iv. T     v. T

In darkened conditions, the light of different wavelengths appears maximally bright in the 480- to 520-nm region, i.e. blue-green. However, in the light-adapted or photopic state the light appears maximally bright in the yellow-green region of wavelength around 560 nm. The Purkinje shift is an important principle and occurs initially in light conditions, when cone function is active. As the luminance decreases, shorter wavelengths become brighter compared to long wavelengths. Cone thresholds can be measured by applying a short bright flash stimuli focused on the central fovea. By desensitising rods with blue light, spectral curves for types of cones can be elicited.[7]
**Difficulty level: 4**

**73**  i. T      ii. F      iii. F      iv. F      v. T

Accommodation occurs independent of convergence, although the two can often act together. When convergence is stopped by the interposition of a base-in prism, contraction of the pupil still occurs during accommodation. The lens shifts anteriorly, increases in curvature and decreases in diameter. Contraction of the ciliary muscle pulls the choroid forwards and releases the tension of the zonular fibres, thereby allowing the lens to form a convex shape. The anterior chamber thus forms a shallower shape. Changes in anterior and posterior capsule tension have also been observed.[8]
   **Difficulty level: 4**

**74**  i. F      ii. F      iii. F      iv. F      v. T

Aqueous humour has been found to contain ascorbic acid, and levels of urea are lower in the aqueous than in the blood. Chloride concentrations have been shown to be higher than in plasma, and both immunoglobulin G and fibronectin levels are lower in concentration compared to plasma. Glucose concentrations are typically 2.7–3.9 mmol/L compared to plasma concentrations, which are 5.6–6.4 mmol/L typically. Sodium and potassium concentrations are similar to plasma, and lactate levels are markedly raised when compared to plasma concentrations. Aqueous humour is secreted by the non-pigmented cells of the ciliary body and is essentially derived from plasma.[7,8]
   **Difficulty level: 3**

**75**  i. T      ii. F      iii. T      iv. T      v. T

The lens of the eye is attached to zonular fibres which attach it to the ciliary processes. The lens epithelium consists of a cuboidal layer of cells and this usually forms a monolayer. The epithelium of the lens has the highest metabolic rate since it actively transports glucose and carbohydrates into the lens, therefore requiring ATP and utilising both glucose and oxygen. The anterior capsule separates the lens from the aqueous humor, and the posterior capsule separates the lens from the vitreous humor.[8]
   **Difficulty level: 2**

**76**   i. T      ii. T      iii. T      iv. F      v. F

Light energy of approximately 50–150 quanta is suggested as a minimum level to perceive light, but only 10%–15% of this actually strikes the retina. However the amount of light required to generate a 'perceived' flash may be higher due to stray light energy from the stimulus and random opening of ion channels. Regeneration of rhodopsin after dark adaptation is around 30 minutes.

The intensity of light energy emitted from a source is measured as luminance, and the units of this are candelas. Lux measures illuminance. One troland equates to a unit of retinal illumination that results when a surface luminance of 1 candela/m$^2$ is viewed through an entrance pupil which measures one square millimetre.[7]

**Difficulty level: 4**


**77**   i. F      ii. T      iii. F      iv. T      v. T

The afferent response of the pupillary light reflex is initiated in the photoreceptors. From the corresponding ganglion cells, fibres enter the optic nerve, pass posteriorly to decussate at the optic chiasm and eventually terminate in the pretectal nucleus. The fibres bypass the lateral geniculate nucleus.

Fibres from the pretectal nucleus then pass through the nucleus of Edinger-Westphal. Fibres pass to the oculomotor nerve nucleus and leave the brainstem via the oculomotor nerve. These fibres synapse in the ciliary ganglion before finally passing through the short ciliary nerves to innervate the sphincter papillae. As a consequence, shining a light stimulus in one eye results in a response in both eyes.[7]

**Difficulty level: 3**


**78**   i. T      ii. T      iii. F      iv. T      v. F

In its resting state, sodium channels in the outer segment of the plasma membrane are kept open. This ensures depolarisation of the cell compared to other cells. Following a light impulse, these channels close, thereby inducing a relative hyperpolarisation. Activation of rhodopsin occurs through the isomerisation of retinol. 11-cis retinal becomes all-trans-retinal. This is then converted to all-trans-retinol, and this does not fit within the rhodopsin transmembrane loops. It detaches from rhodopsin and is taken up by the RPE cell, where it is converted to 11-cis retinol and binds to cellular retinal binding pro-

tein (CRALBP). Rhodopsin is synthesised in the endoplasmic reticulum and Golgi apparatus of the inner and not outer segments of the photoreceptor.[7]
**Difficulty level: 4**

**79**  i. T    ii. F    iii. F    iv. F    v. T

The electroretinogram (ERG) is a useful investigation for the assessment of retinal function. The early receptor potential can be detected in eyes where the inner retina has been destroyed but the outer retina is intact. One clinical scenario where this can occur is in a central retinal artery occlusion. The negative a-wave is generated by hyperpolarisation in the photoreceptor inner segments. The a1 component of this originates from the cones and the a2 component from the rods. The b-wave is generated from bipolar cells, and the slow-rising c-wave originates from the retinal pigment epithelium.[7]
**Difficulty level: 4**

**80**  i. F    ii. T    iii. T    iv. F    v. F

The visual evoked potential (VEP) records electrical activity from the occipital cortex after light is presented to the retina. A total of usually six electrodes are placed around the left and right occipital cortex. Several types of VEP can be induced, including flash, flash-pattern, pattern-onset and pattern-reversal VEPs. A pattern-flash VEP can be induced by presenting a black-and-white chequerboard stimulus. The flash VEP arises from the V2 area of the cortex, whereas the pattern VEP arises from the V1 area of the cortex. Clinically, this test is very useful for the assessment of optic nerve dysfunction.[7]
**Difficulty level: 5**

**81**  i. F    ii. T    iii. F    iv. T    v. F

The lacrimal gland is a tubuloacinar gland and is composed of many lobules separated by interstitial fibrovascular septae. Histologically, the lacrimal gland appears very similar to the parotid gland. Each tubuloacinar unit consists of single layers of cuboidal or columnar cells. A layer of myoepithelial cells surrounds each acinus. The secretion of the lacrimal gland is mainly proteinaceous, although many of the granules contain mucopolysaccharides. Lacrimal secretion contains high concentrations of lysozymes, lactoferrin, β-lysine and immunoglobulin A (IgA). Lymphocytes and mast cells are also released, and these serve to protect the ocular surface from pathogens.[7]
**Difficulty level: 4**

**82**    i.   T      ii.   F      iii.   T      iv.   T      v.   F

The striate cortex regions V1–V5 are extremely specialised. All of the cells in area V5 respond to motion in the visual system and are directionally selective. None of these cells are colour specific. Cells in area V4 are colour wavelength specific but some are recognised as being involved in shape detection. Cells in area V3 are also implicated in form and shape detection. The V2 area is implicated in motion and colour detection. Positron emission tomography (PET) and functional magnetic resonance imaging (FMRI) have been shown useful in identifying these areas, mapping increases in cerebral blood flow.[7]

**Difficulty level: 5**

**83**    i.   F      ii.   F      iii.   T      iv.   F      v.   F

In the Snellen chart, each letter has five elements. Each element has a minimum angle of resolution of 1 minute of arc when looking at the 6/6 line from 1 metre. The Snellen visual acuity scale represents the reciprocal of the minimum angle of resolution. Therefore, when looking from 6 metres at the 6/24 line of the Snellen chart, 4 minutes of arc is required for the element to be resolved.[9]

**Difficulty level: 2**

**84**    i.   T      ii.   T      iii.   T      iv.   F      v.   F

Contrast sensitivity is a measure of the minimal amount of contrast required to distinguish a test object. The Pelli-Robson contrast sensitivity letter chart is viewed at 1 metre and consists of rows of letters of equal size but with decreasing contrast of 0.15 log units for every group of three letters. Ishihara charts test colour vision.[1]

**Difficulty level: 3**

**85**    i.   F      ii.   F      iii.   F      iv.   T      v.   T

Visual acuity decreases with increased refractive error and retinal eccentricity.[7]

**Difficulty level: 3**

**86**    i.   F      ii.   F      iii.   F      iv.   F      v.   F

Colour is perceived at the cortical level. The three cone opsins have maximum absorbance at differing wavelengths, namely 425, 530 and 560 nm. Blue cones are the most scarce. Colour perceived is dependent upon luminance. Rods are not involved in colour vision.[7]

**Difficulty level: 2**

87   i. T      ii. F      iii. F      iv. T      v. T

Stereopsis is not present at birth. It first appears at 4 months of age and continues to develop through the early years of life. Stereopsis is poor beyond 20 degrees from the fovea. The Lang test is a random-dot stereogram. The degree of stereopsis is measured by altering the degree of displacement between the random dots.[9]

**Difficulty level: 3**

88   i. T      ii. F      iii. F      iv. T      v. T

Panum's area is the range of angular disparities over which vision is single and fused. It is possible to fuse greater disparities in the horizontal meridian than the vertical, and therefore Panum's area forms an ellipse. Too large an angle of disparity leads to diplopia. The area varies with the form and eccentricity of the target but is not dependent on size or colour.[7]

**Difficulty level: 4**

89   i. T      ii. F      iii. F      iv. T      v. F

The parvocellular pathway conveys information on colour and fine detail as well as being important for spatial discrimination. The parvocellular pathway has slower responses, slower speed of conduction and smaller receptive fields compared to the magnocellular pathway.[7]

**Difficulty level: 4**

90   i. T      ii. T      iii. T      iv. T      v. F

The magnocellular pathway is most responsive to motion, flicker and light detection. The magnocellular pathway contains ganglion cells with large dendritic trees contributing to the large receptive fields of this pathway. The ganglion cells in the magnocellular pathway demonstrate non-linear spatial summation and respond in a transient manner. The parvocellular pathway demonstrates more sustained responses and linear spatial summation.[7]

**Difficulty level: 4**

**91**   i. T     ii. F     iii. F     iv. F     v. T

Optokinetic nystagmus is a reflex to prolonged full-field visual motion such as a rotating drum. It is a physiological process supplementing the vestibular ocular reflex to stabilise vision. It is different from vestibular nystagmus and therefore does not involve the semicircular canals.[10]

**Difficulty level: 4**

**92**   i. F     ii. F     iii. T     iv. T     v. T

In Horner's syndrome both the upper lid and lower lid are involved. Paresis of the lower tarsal muscle causes the lower lid to rise, thereby narrowing the palpebral aperture. Anhydrosis of the affected side of the face only occurs if the lesion involves the sympathetic pathway proximal to the bifurcation of the common carotid artery, since the sudomotor fibres travel with the external carotid artery.[10]

**Difficulty level: 3**

**93**   i. F     ii. F     iii. T     iv. T     v. F

Eighty per cent of cases of Adie's tonic pupil are unilateral at presentation but tend to become bilateral at a rate of 4% per year. There is a female predilection (70% vs 30%). It is thought to be due to aberrant regeneration of parasympathetic fibres in the short posterior ciliary nerves after damage to the ciliary ganglion.[10]

**Difficulty level: 3**

**94**   i. F     ii. T     iii. F     iv. F     v. T

The electroretinogram measures the electrical mass response of the entire retina to light stimulation. The a-wave is a negative deflection produced by photoreceptors. It is followed by a corneal positive deflection, the b-wave, generated by the Müller cells. With the standard bright white flash, a mixed rod-cone response is generated. The rods have poor temporal resolution and are therefore unable to respond to a 30-Hz stimulus.[7]

**Difficulty level: 3**

**95**   i. T   ii. F   iii. F   iv. F   v. T

As the EOG is a measure of retinal pigment epithelial activity, it cannot distinguish between cone and rod dysfunction or between optic nerve and macula disease. In the case of Best's vitelliform dystrophy, the electroretinogram (ERG) is normal but the EOG light rise is markedly reduced.[7]
   **Difficulty level: 3**

**96**   i. T   ii. T   iii. T   iv. F   v. T

VEPs are a useful objective test in children where subjective information may be difficult to obtain. Optic nerve dysfunction characteristically produces a delay in P100 (characteristic positive component approximately 100 ms after presentation of a reversing chequered box) often associated with an amplitude reduction.[7]
   **Difficulty level: 3**

**97**   i. T   ii. T   iii. T   iv. T   v. T

Dark adaptation curves form the basis of the duplicity theory, which states that above certain thresholds of illuminance the cone system is mainly responsible for mediating vision and below this threshold the rod system is more important.[7]
   **Difficulty level: 3**

**98**   i. F   ii. T   iii. F   iv. F   v. F

In light-near dissociation the pupils demonstrate a better response to accommodative targets than light stimuli. It is associated with Argyll Robertson pupils, Adie's tonic pupil, dorsal midbrain syndrome and aberrant degeneration of the 3rd cranial nerve.[10]
   **Difficulty level: 3**

**99**   i. T   ii. T   iii. T   iv. T   v. F

With Argyll Robertson pupils, there is not a tonic response to pupil dilation after the near target has been removed – this helps to distinguish them from Adie's pupil. The Argyll Robertson pupil is associated with neurosyphilis, diabetes, multiple sclerosis, sarcoidosis and alcoholism.[10]
   **Difficulty level: 3**

**100**   i. F      ii. T      iii. F      iv. F      v. T

Oxytocin is structurally similar to vasopressin and can therefore reduce urine production slightly. Its effects include uterine contraction in the second and third stages of labour, and the 'breastfeeding reflex', whereby breast milk is released into the subareolar sinuses when the nipples are stimulated.[2]

**Difficulty level: 4**


# References

1   Kanski JJ. *Clinical Ophthalmology – a systematic approach*. 6th ed. Edinburgh: Butterworth Heinemann Elsevier; 2007. (**q51**) pp. 285–6, (**q84**) p. 20.

2   Guyton AC, Hall J. *Textbook of Medical Physiology*. 11th ed. Edinburgh: Saunders Elsevier; 2006. (**q51**) pp. 875–6, (**q54**) p. 188, (**q55**) pp. 72–3, (**q56**) p. 74, (**q58**) p. 168, (**q59**) pp. 561–3, (**q60**) pp. 598–9, (**q65**) pp. 121–2, (**q100**) pp. 924–5.

3   Olson JH, Erie JC, Bakri SJ. Nutritional supplementation and age-related macular degeneration. *Semin Ophthalmol*. 2011; **26**(3): 131–6 (**q52**).

4   Denniston A, Murray P. *Oxford Handbook of Ophthalmology*. Oxford: Oxford University Press; 2006. (**q53**) p. 473.

5   Colledge NR, Walker BR, Ralston SH. *Davidson's Principles and Practice of Medicine*. 21st ed. Edinburgh: Churchill Livingstone Elsevier; 2010. (**q57**) pp. 1022–7.

6   Snell R, Lemp M. *Clinical Anatomy of the Eye*. 2nd ed. Malden: Blackwell Science; 1998. (**q61**) pp. 120–1, (**q62**) pp. 120–1, (**q63**) pp. 157–9, (**q64**) pp. 191, 196.

7   Forrester J, Dick A, McMenamin A, *et al*. *The Eye: basic sciences in practice*. 2nd ed. Philadelphia: Saunders Elsevier; 2007. (**q61**) p. 176, (**q66**) pp. 234–5, (**q71**) pp. 235–8, (**q72**) pp. 239–42, (**q74**) pp. 187–8, (**q76**) pp. 228–30, (**q77**) p. 232, (**q78**) pp. 216–17, (**q79**) pp. 238–40, (**q80**) pp. 238–42, (**q81**) pp. 84–6, (**q82**) pp. 255–60, (**q85**) p. 228, (**q86**) p. 241, (**q88**) p. 252, (**q89, q90**) p. 254, (**q94, q95, q96**) pp. 238–9, (**q97**) p. 226.

8   Kaufman P, Alm A. *Adler's Physiology of the Eye – clinical application*. 10th ed. Philadelphia: Mosby Elsevier; 2003. (**q67**) pp. 843–5, (**q68**) pp. 323–8, (**q69**) pp. 33–9, (**q70**) pp. 132–3, (**q73**) pp. 197–204, (**74**) pp. 237–44, (**q75**) pp. 118–37.

9   Madge S, Kersey J, Hawker M, *et al*. *Clinical Techniques in Ophthalmology*. Edinburgh: Churchill Livingstone; 2006. (**q83**) p. 99, (**q87**) p. 165.

10  Kline LB. *Neuro-Ophthalmology Review Manual*. 6th ed. New Jersey: Slack; 2007. (**q91**) p. 76, (**q92**) pp. 133–5, (**q93**) pp. 131–2, (**q98, q99**) p. 132.

# 3. Biochemistry and cell biology FRCOphth answers

1   **D**   The ciliary body forms part of the blood-aqueous barrier. Ciliary body blood flow is typically under autonomic control.[1]
**Difficulty level: 2**

2   **A**   The retina consists of approximately 20% lipid. These are predominantly phospholipids which play an important role in the regulation of rhodopsin.[1]
**Difficulty level: 3**

3   **D**   The CD1 antigen is thought to play a role in T-cell receptor signalling. Fibronectin, ICAM-1 and CD44 antigen play significant roles in cell adhesion.[1]
**Difficulty level: 4**

4   **C**   Types IV, VII, IX and XV collagen, along with lamina densa and hemidesmosomes, achieve adhesion of the epithelial basement membrane and Bowman's layer.[1] Cadherins are a type of transmembrane and are responsible for cell-to-cell adhesion. E-cadherin is the epithelial form. Fodrin is a cytoskeletal protein and it is thought that there are important changes in these molecules that precede actin rearrangement.[1]
**Difficulty level: 4**

5   **C**   The ciliary body contains a significant proportion of $\alpha_2$ receptors. Stimulation of these presynaptic receptors results in a decrease in intraocular pressure through increased outflow, contraction of Müller's muscle and constriction of conjunctival and episcleral vessels.[1]
**Difficulty level: 4**

6   **D**   They appear to have low levels of microtubules. Microtubules form cylindrical shapes within cells and play an important role in endcytosis and cytoplasmic movement of organelles. This, along with the high levels of actin, means that trabecular meshwork cells are efficient at endocytosis and contractility.[1]
**Difficulty level: 3**

**7  C**  A G protein is a transmembrane protein to which a drug binds. G proteins are signalling proteins. They interact with secondary messengers such as cyclic AMP, inositol phosphates and cyclic GMP.[2]
**Difficulty level: 3**

**8  C**  Calcium is stored within discrete compartments within the cell cytoplasm.[3,4]
**Difficulty level: 3**

**9  C**  Clathrin-coated pits are usually restricted to an area of the plasma membrane, and are related to the underlying cytoskeletal actin arrangement. Latruculin B is thought to play an important role in the relaxation of actin, thereby allowing the pits to move.[1]
**Difficulty level: 3**

**10  B**  Photoreceptor turnover, the recycling use of the same photoreceptor, occurs in a diurnal manner. Complete renewal of the rod outer segment, whereby a new segment is created, takes 9–10 days, and they utilise glucose in both an anaerobic and aerobic manner.[1]
**Difficulty level: 3**

**11  C**  Desmosomal junctions are approximately 20 nm in width between cells. GAP junctions are composed of connexons (a cylindrical form of six connexin proteins) which connect across the intercellular space. ICAM-1 is not present.[1]
**Difficulty level: 4**

**12  A**  IL-12 is involved in stimulating the Th1 response, GM-CSF for monocyte maturation and IFN-γ for macrophage activation.[1]
**Difficulty level: 4**

**13  C**  Chromatin in its condensed form is not a good template for transcription. Usually chromatin remodelling is required before transcription can proceed.[3]
**Difficulty level: 4**

**14  A**  Cytokines may also be effective at low concentrations.[3]
**Difficulty level: 4**

**15  D**  Catalase acts as an $H_2O_2$ degrading enzyme. Vitamins A and E are free radical scavengers.[3]
**Difficulty level: 3**

**16 A** Leukotriene $B_4$ ($LTB_4$) is chemotactic leukotriene and acts as a neutrophil. Thromboxane $A_2$ is a platelet aggregator. Prostaglandin $E_2$ is involved in mucosal protection, smooth muscle relaxation and a variety of other metabolic effects such as the inhibition of lipolysis. Phospholipase $A_2$ is an enzyme involved in the formation of arachidonic acid.[5]
**Difficulty level: 2**

**17 D** Histamine type 2 receptors affect the release of gastric acid.[3,5]
**Difficulty level: 3**

**18 D** A drug showing both antagonistic and agonistic properties is known as a partial agonist. At a very high concentration, a partial agonist will behave as an antagonist as it interferes with true agonists docking with the receptor.[5]
**Difficulty level: 3**

**19 B** Flow cytometry can be used to identify phenotypically different cells. Western blotting may be used to detect proteins, and Northern blotting is used for the detection of specific RNA samples.[1]
**Difficulty level: 3**

**20 A** MIP26 is a lens fibre-specific junctional protein, and is heavily involved in intercellular communication. MIP is one of the aquaporins, and it is also postulated that MIP26 helps pump water out of the lens. Mutations in the gene coding for MIP26 result in cataracts in murine models. Calpactins are inhibitors of the calpains (which are neural endopeptidases). Crystallins are found in the lens epithelium and cortex, and act as substrates for the endopeptidases.[1]
**Difficulty level: 3**

**21 C** The vitreous retards the bulk flow of fluid.[1]
**Difficulty level: 3**

**22 D** Steroids are synthesised in the smooth endoplasmic reticulum.[4]
**Difficulty level: 4**

**23 A** The cytoplasm is a very viscous medium, and microfilaments are thought to play an important role. Microfilaments also insert into junctional complexes, thereby playing a role in structural integrity.[1]
**Difficulty level: 3**

**24 D** Hypertension can occur in around 50% of patients, whereas nephrotoxicity occurs very frequently in patients given this immunosuppressant

drug. Over a prolonged period of administration, interstitial fibrosis and tubular atrophy may occur. Caution should be exercised in concurrent use with other nephrotoxic agents such as aminoglycosides and antimicrobials.[5]
**Difficulty level: 3**

**25 A** Adherens-type junctions are desmosomes and form connections of 20 nm in width. Zonula adherens are a type of desmosome and are a ring around the apex of the cell.[1]
**Difficulty level: 4**

**26 D** Immunohistochemistry uses specific constituents of cells' pathological identification. One example could be the presence of smooth muscle actin in leiomyomas. Using the peroxidise/antiperoxidase technique, the metabolic activity of the cell can be identified. Fixation of the antigen using glutaraldehyde alone is not very effective, but exposing sections to microwaves or high-pressure steam can lead to better preservation. The technique is useful for malignant lymphoma, for example.[1]
**Difficulty level: 4**

**27 B** The choroid has no recognised lymphoid system.[1]
**Difficulty level: 3**

**28 C** Retinal pigment epithelial (RPE) cells when under stress secrete IL-1. Their turnover is very slow, and they have been shown to express CD38. GLUT-1 and -3 are types of $Na^+$-independent facilitated-diffusion glucose transporters: GLUT-1 is located in all cells, and GLUT-3 is present in most cells. GLUT-3 transports glucose from the cerebrospinal fluid across the plasma membranes of neuronal cells.[1]
**Difficulty level: 3**

**29 D** The retinal vessels are impermeable to molecules greater than 20 000 Da.[1]
**Difficulty level: 3**

**30 A** The sclera contains a few fibroblasts but is otherwise acellular. The distributions of collagen types I and III are irregular and this helps give an opaque appearance.[1]
**Difficulty level: 3**

## References

1  Forrester J, Dick A, McMenamin A, *et al. The Eye: basic sciences in practice.* 2nd
   ed. Philadelphia: Saunders Elsevier; 2007. (**q1**) pp. 187–90, (**q2**) pp. 206–10,
   (**q3**) pp. 211–15, (**q4**) pp. 178–80, (**q5**) pp. 284–6, (**q6**) pp. 195–6, (**q9, q11**)
   pp. 160–1, (**q10**) pp. 208–9, (**q12**) pp. 318–19, (**q19**) pp. 432–3, (**q20**) pp. 196–9,
   (**q21**) pp. 205–6, (**q23, q25**) pp. 160–2, (**q26**) pp. 432–3, (**q27**) pp. 191–3, (**q28**)
   pp. 213–16, (**q29**) pp. 210–16, (**q30**) pp. 187–90.
2  Winstanley P, Walley T. *Pharmacology.* 1st ed. Edinburgh: Churchill Livingstone;
   1996. (**q7**) p. 10.
3  Baynes J, Dominiczak M. *Medical Biochemistry.* 2nd ed. Philadelphia: Elsevier;
   2005. (**q8**) pp. 35, 96, (**q13**) p. 466, (**q14**) pp. 508–9, (**q15**) pp. 502–3, (**q17**) p. 123.
4  Devlin T. *Textbook of Biochemistry.* 6th ed. New York: Wiley-Liss; 2006. (**q8, q22**)
   pp. 14–15.
5  Waller D, Renwick A, Hillier K. *Medical Pharmacology and Therapeutics.* Edinburgh:
   Saunders Elsevier; 2001. (**q16**) pp. 305–6, (**q17**) pp. 64–5, (**q18**) p. 14, (**q24**)
   pp. 379–81.

# 3. Biochemistry and cell biology ICO answers

**31**   i. F       ii. T       iii. F       iv. T       v. F

A decrease in insulin has a number of effects, both on carbohydrate metabolism
as well as protein and fat metabolism. There is an increase in glycogenolysis
and gluconeogenesis which dually result in an increase in liver output of glucose. This secondarily results in a glycosuria and osmotic diuresis, which in
turns leads to a depletion of sodium and water. The net result of this is the
symptom of thirst brought about by dehydration. Hyperventilation results
from an increase in plasma free fatty acids, and acetone odours on the breath
are brought about by an increase in ketogenesis resulting in ketonaemia.[1]
   **Difficulty level: 3**

**32**    i. T      ii. F      iii. T      iv. T      v. F

NF-κB, AP-1, c-Jun and c-Fos are transcription factors. GLUT-1 is a glucose transporter. Following intracellular signalling, transcription factors are activated, resulting in the formation of proteins.[2]
   **Difficulty level: 2**

**33**    i. T      ii. T      iii. T      iv. F      v. F

The stages of the cell cycle can be divided into four phases (although in some literature, interphase encompasses $G_0$, $G_1$, S and $G_2$ phases). In the S phase, the chromosomal DNA is duplicated, which is followed by $G_2$ phase and then M phase in which mitosis occurs leading to the division of cell organelles into two progeny cells. In M phase a number of important events occur. These include nuclear membrane disintegration, chromosomal alignment along the equator of the cell, and mitotic spindle formation. In a human fibroblast cell the M phase lasts about 1 hour. Cells present in phase $G_0$ tend to have a low metabolic rate and low rates of protein transcription.[3]
   **Difficulty level: 3**

**34**    i. T      ii. T      iii. T      iv. F      v. T

Intraocular pressure is created by aqueous humor production and resorption through the trabecular meshwork. It is therefore affected by anterior chamber anatomy and episcleral venous pressure. Whilst the measurement reading of IOP is affected by hormonal influences, it is not affected by arterial pressure directly.[2]
   **Difficulty level: 4**

**35**    i. T      ii. T      iii. F      iv. F      v. T

Within haemoglobin, of which the haem group is almost insoluble in water but soluble when bound to globin, oxygen and carbon dioxide compete for the same binding sites, and thus an increase in carbon dioxide concentration results in a decrease in affinity for oxygen. Haemoglobin requires all iron atoms to be in the FeII oxygenation state, and it usually contains four atoms. Four polypeptide chains exist but there are no disulphide bonds present. When oxygenated, sickle-cell haemoglobin is more soluble than normal adult haemoglobin. Fetal human haemoglobin differs from adult haemoglobin and contains two alpha and two gamma units.[4]
   **Difficulty level: 4**

**36**   i. T      ii. F      iii. F      iv. F      v. T

Mitochondria are typically ova-shaped organelles, and consist of a two-membrane system, which are folded internally to form cristae. Mitochondriae contain a number of functions, including acting as a calcium store. Mitochondria have their own DNA but no histones. Transmission of genetic material in mitochondria is purely maternal. The aspartate/glutamate transport system is present within mitochondria, along with the malate/citrate and ornithine/citrulline systems.[2]
   **Difficulty level: 4**

**37**   i. F      ii. F      iii. T      iv. T      v. T

Pyruvate is essential in energy production and can be formed from glycolysis of glucose. Pyruvate may then be reduced to lactate, by carboxylation to oxyaloacetate, through transamination form alanine, or form acetyl-CoA through oxidative decarboxylation. The proportion of transformation to these various groups depends upon the metabolic state of the cell.
   Acetyl-CoA is generated from free fatty acids through β-oxidation as well, and through deamination of amino acids. It is a large, hydrophilic molecule. Acetyl-CoA has an important function, acting as a feedback inhibitor for pyruvate dehydrogenase, and dihydrolipoyl transacetylase is essential for the transfer of the acetyl group to coenzyme A.[3]
   **Difficulty level: 5**

**38**   i. T      ii. F      iii. T      iv. F      v. T

Stimulating hormones usually bind to the cell and instigate a variety of secondary messenger systems. Cyclic AMP and GMP are often involved, along with phosphatidylinositol-triphosphatase ($PIP_3$). The secondary messenger pathway has an amplification effect, with one reaction generating a cascade of other reactions. The intracellular second messengers activate specific kinases that initiate a cascade of phosphorylation and dephosphorylation reactions. Stimulation of adenylate cyclase generates cAMP which activates protein kinase C. The effects of cyclic AMP are terminated when hydrolysed by phosphodiesterase. Transcription factors are activated by protein kinase A which has catalysed the phosphorylation of a cAMP response element binding protein. This activated binding protein binds to a specific promoter region of a gene and initiates transcription.[3]
   **Difficulty level: 5**

**39**   i.  F      ii.  T      iii.  F      iv.  T      v.  T

Vitamin A, also known as retinol, is a fat-soluble vitamin commonly found in liver, fish oils and dairy products. Other fat-soluble vitamins include D, E and K. Vitamin E is known as tocopherol, and a deficiency in this can lead to infertility. Thiamine is a water-soluble vitamin and a deficiency of this can lead to a condition known as beriberi, which can result in altered cardiac function, as well as Wernicke's encephalopathy. Vitamin $B_{12}$ is synthesised by micro-organisms and is present in meat. Ascorbic acid is essential in the synthesis of collagen, where it acts as a coenzyme for both proline hydroxylase and lysyl hydroxylase.[4]

**Difficulty level: 3**

**40**   i.  F      ii.  F      iii.  T      iv.  T      v.  T

Various mutations can affect biochemical pathways with resultant conditions. Homocysteinuria affects the amino acid methionine, and it does this by acting upon the cystathione synthetase enzyme. Tyrosinaemia is a defect of tyrosine metabolism; type 1 affects fumarylacetoacetate hydrolase, and type 2 affects tyrosine aminotransferase. Albinism is a tyrosinase enzyme defect acting upon the amino acid tyrosine. There are many types of glycogen storage diseases of which glucose 6-phosphatase deficiency typically affects the liver, kidney and intestine. A defect in phenylalanine hydroxylase results in phenylketonuria (PKU).[4]

**Difficulty level: 4**

**41**   i.  F      ii.  T      iii.  T      iv.  F      v.  T

Sodium independent facilitated diffusion transporters (GLUTs) are ubiquitously expressed in mammalian cells. They are principally responsible for the movement of glucose from the blood into cells. GLUT-1 is present in all tissues, including erythrocytes. GLUT-2 is present in high concentrations in the pancreas, and has a high affinity for glucose. GLUT-3 is present in most cells including the brain. GLUT-5 is important for fructose absorption. The conversion of glucose to fructose 1,6-bisphosphate is the first step of glycolysis, and the enzymes involved in this step are glucokinase/hexokinase and then phosphofructokinase-1. Glycolysis helps generate a limited amount of ATP.[4]

**Difficulty level: 4**

**42**    i. T        ii. T        iii. F        iv. T        v. F

A number of tissue proteoglycans exist, with specific roles. Collagen type II is present within the stroma, and aggrecan is a tissue proteoglycan present in cartilage and important for structural support. Thrombospondins are a group of molecules secreted by endothelial cells and are thought to be involved in the regulation of angiogenesis. Tissue inhibitors of matrix metalloproteinases (TIMPs) are important in tissue remodelling. Fibrillin is found in the vitreous.[2]

**Difficulty level: 3**

**43**    i. T        ii. T        iii. F        iv. F        v. T

The mitochondria play an extremely important role within a cell, accounting for approximately 90% of the adenosine-triphosphate (ATP) required by the cell. They are usually up to 1 micron in diameter and up to 7 microns in length. Exercise results in an increase in mitochondria within skeletal muscle. They play an important role in ageing, and cytochrome c is an initiator in programmed cell death. Mitochondria also play a role in their own replication, and electron microscopy shows that mitochondria contain genetic information for 13 mitochondrial proteins and some RNAs.[3]

**Difficulty level: 3**

**44**    i. F        ii. F        iii. F        iv. T        v. F

Nuclear chromatin consists of DNA and protein. This condenses to form chromosomes during cell division. Euchromatin is less densely packed than heterochromatin. The nucleolus is essentially composed of RNA and fibrillar material. It is the site of ribosomal RNA synthesis.[2]

**Difficulty level: 4**

**45**    i. F        ii. T        iii. T        iv. F        v. F

Lysosomes are responsible for intracellular digestion of both intracellular and extracellular substances. They contain a variety of enzymes such as collagenase and hyaluronidase. There are a variety of other enzymes contained within the lysosome, including sulfatases, phosphatases and other lipid hydrolysing and nucleic acid hydrolysing enzymes. They maintain an acidic pH of approximately 5. Lysosomes are involved in the process of endocytosis, in which material from the external environment is taken into the cell and encapsulated into membrane-bound vesicles. Lysosomes are also very involved in the hydrolysis of cellular components – a process known as autophagy.[3]

**Difficulty level: 2**

**46**  i. T     ii. T     iii. F     iv. F     v. F

The cornea is a six-cell layer of which the cells express fibronectin, laminin and collagen. Zonula occludens are absent, whereas hemidesmosomes are present. The corneal stroma contains no hyaluronic acid. Stromal collagen type II accounts for 50%–55% of collagen, and types IV and VII collagen are also present and are in contact with the epithelial and endothelial cell layers. Type V collagen accounts for approximately 10% of the total collagen present in the stroma. The collagen fibres typically are arranged at oblique angles to each other, but have a uniform thickness and this is important for the purposes of light diffraction and transmission.[2]

**Difficulty level: 3**

**47**  i. F     ii. T     iii. F     iv. T     v. F

The ciliary body plays an important role in maintaining the concentration of various electrolytes in the anterior chamber. There are a number of anti-oxidant and detoxification systems present, and the ciliary body is abundant with catalase, superoxide dismutase and glutathione peroxidise types 1 and 2. The main role of type 1 is to reduce oxidised glutathione. Hydrogen peroxide is present in the aqueous humor and it is reduced to $H_2O$ by glutathione secreted by the ciliary epithelium. Melatonin acts as an $H_2O_2$ scavenger as well. Prostaglandin secretion is increased in trauma and inflammation.[2]

**Difficulty level: 3**

**48**  i. T     ii. F     iii. F     iv. T     v. T

Three types of crystallins, α, β and γ, make up approximately 90% of the water-soluble proteins of the lens. Alpha (α) crystallins also trap other proteins and filaments. A number of cytoskeletal elements are present in the lens, including actin, vimentin and spectrin. Vimentin is the major intermediate filament in the lens cell. Cytokeratins are not found in the adult lens. The lens capsule contains type IV collagen and heparin sulphate, and this serves to act as a diffusion barrier for the lens. Fibronectin is present mainly in the anterior capsule, whereas tenascin is present in the posterior capsule.[2]

**Difficulty level: 3**

**49**    i. F      ii. T      iii. F      iv. F      v. T

The vitreous is made up of approximately 98% water, with the rest being made up of macromolecules. Collagen fibrils are filled with glycosaminoglycans between them, and this has the effect of reducing further diffraction of light. With age, a process known as vitreous syneresis occurs whereby hyaluronic acid is degraded into smaller molecules. Type VI collagen is present in the vitreous and may play a structural role. Hyalocytes are present in the vitreous cavity and produce hyaluronic acid in the gel. There is no regeneration of collagen in the vitreous with age.[2]

**Difficulty level: 3**

**50**    i. T      ii. T      iii. T      iv. T      v. F

A variety of retinal neurotransmitters and neuromodulators are present in the human retina, and exert a number of excitatory and inhibitory roles. Neurotransmitters have a rapid action at the synaptic junction, whereas neuromodulators have a much longer action. Glycine and GABA are examples of typical inhibitory transmitters. Glutamate is present and acts on photoreceptors, as well as serotonin. Substance P acts on both amacrine and ganglion cells. Neurotensin acts on amacrine cells, whereas β-endorphin acts upon amacrine and ganglion cells rather than photoreceptor cells.[2]

**Difficulty level: 4**

**51**    i. F      ii. F      iii. F      iv. F      v. T

Adrenergic and cholinergic receptors are present both within the iris and also ciliary body. Muscarinic receptors are also present in the ciliary epithelium. The majority of the receptors in the ciliary body are α2. Beta-2 (β2) receptors account for more than 90% of all β receptors. Stimulation, rather than blockade of β2 receptors, leads to an increase in aqueous secretion via the activation of adenylate cyclase. Adrenergic receptors are present in the ciliary body, regulating intraocular pressure via the adenylate cyclase system.[2]

**Difficulty level: 3**

**52**    i. T      ii. T      iii. F      iv. T      v. T

The cell membrane is an essential biological membrane and acts to separate the cytoplasm from the external environment. Fungi, bacteria and some plants also possess a cell membrane. It consists of a predominantly phospholipid bilayer, although there are proteins which are adherent to both surfaces and these play an important role in cell signalling. Three main types of lipids exist – phospholipids, glycolipids and cholesterols. The membrane can act as a selective barrier to allow molecules to enter and exit the cell, and they exhibit polarity. Cell membranes, in addition, play an important role in cell-to-cell adhesion.[5]

**Difficulty level: 2**

**53**  i.  T        ii.  F        iii.  F        iv.  T        v.  F

Succinyl CoA is an essential component of the Krebs cycle, whereby carbohydrates are broken down to generate carbon dioxide and water, along with energy for the cell. Pyruvate is an essential component, and one turn of the Krebs cycle generates 1 ATP molecule, with two turns required per molecule of glucose and thus two ATP produced. The total amount of ATP produced by breakdown of glucose through glycolysis, the Krebs cycle and β-oxidation is approximately 30. The regulation of the Krebs cycle is due to substrate availability. Citrate is important for feedback inhibition, rather than pyruvate, as it inhibits phosphofructokinase.[6]

**Difficulty level: 3**

**54**  i.  T        ii.  F        iii.  T        iv.  F        v.  T

Vascular endothelial growth factor (VEGF) has received a great deal of attention from the scientific community in recent years. VEGF has been shown to stimulate angiogenesis as well as the mitotic rate of endothelial cells. It aids the creation of vessel lumen and creates capillary fenestrations. Due to these effects it can be said to promote neovascularisation and is overexpressed in certain pathological states in the eye, such as age-related macular degeneretion and other proliferative retinopathies. VEGF may be upregulated by a cellular response to hypoxia via an upregulation of hypoxia inducible factor (HIF).[7]

**Difficulty level: 2**

**55**  i.  T        ii.  F        iii.  T        iv.  T        v.  T

Vitamin A is essential for corneal and conjunctival health, and it is required for epithelial keratin expression, as well as glycoprotein synthesis. A deficiency of vitamin A results in poor corneal wound healing and, clinically, Bitot's spots and punctate epithelial erosions. Vitamin A is essential for the inhibition of proteolytic enzymes.[2]

**Difficulty level: 3**

**56**   **i.** F      **ii.** F      **iii.** T      **iv.** T      **v.** T

There are a number of natural oxidant/antioxidant systems within the lens and these help to maintain the internal milieu. Cells decrease cytoskeletal organisation with age, with a decrease in enzymatic activity. Production of β- and γ-crystallin increases with age. Other changes that can be seen include an increase in water content, and vacuolation within the lens fibers. The lens naturally contains high concentrations of glutathione and this prevents ascorbic acid being oxidised. Ascorbic acid, when oxidised, interacts with lens crystallin and promotes crystallin glycation and hence further cataract formation.[2]

**Difficulty level: 4**

**57**   **i.** T      **ii.** F      **iii.** F      **iv.** T      **v.** T

The blood-retinal barrier is essential in maintaining the retinal microenvironment, and is maintained by tight junctions. Retinal vessels are impermeable to molecules larger than 20 000 Da. Nitric oxide acts as a vasodilator and helps to dilate retinal vasculature; endothelin helps to constrict blood vessels. Pericytes possess contractile properties that regulate bloodflow, and have high-affinity receptors IGF-1 and IGF-2. These may be involved in glucose transport and protein synthesis.[2]

**Difficulty level: 3**

**58**   **i.** T      **ii.** T      **iii.** T      **iv.** T      **v.** F

Rod photoreceptor outer segments turn over rapidly. The passage of rhodopsin insertion into the disc plasma membrane of the RPE is complex. Glycosylation of rhodopsin occurs through a number of steps and can be inhibited by tunicamycin. Rod outer segment disc shedding occurs in a diurnal manner, and phagocytosis of disc outer segment occurs in the retinal pigment epithelium. Cone outer segments are generally more stable and turnover is slower than rod outer segments.[2]

**Difficulty level: 3**

**59**    i. T        ii. T        iii. F        iv. F        v. T

The initial step in the visual impulse is the activation of rhodopsin from the isomerisation of retinol. 11-cis-retinal is converted to all-trans-retinal in the presence of light, which via a G-protein coupled receptor activates a signal transduction cascade resulting in hyperpolarisation of the cell.

Subsequently, all-trans-retinal becomes converted to all-trans-retinol, which does not fit within the rhodopsin molecule and is released. It is taken up by the retinal pigment epithelium (RPE). In dark adapted conditions this molecule is converted to 11-cis-retinol and this binds cellular retinal binding protein (CRALBP). Vitamin A deficiency results in poor vision in low levels of light illumination. When a molecule of rhodopsin is activated, an amplification cascade is generated, leading to the opening and closure of many sodium channels, resulting in a change in the resting potential of the photoreceptor.[2]

**Difficulty level: 4**


**60**    i. T        ii. F        iii. T        iv. T        v. T

Gamma aminobutyric acid (GABA) is an inhibitory neurotransmitter and is present in high concentrations of the retina, whereas L-aspartate and acetylcholine are excitatory neurotransmitters. Glycine is an inhibitory neurotransmitter. Dopamine is thought to be an inhibitory neurotransmitter.[2,8]

**Difficulty level: 3**


## References

1  Beckett G, Walker S, Rae P, *et al. Clinical Biochemistry*. 8th ed. New York: Wiley-Blackwell; 2007. (**q31**) p. 97.

2  Forrester J, Dick A, McMenamin A, *et al. The Eye: basic sciences in practice*. 2nd ed. Philadelphia: Saunders Elsevier; 2007. (**q32**) p. 169, (**q34**) pp. 192–3, (**q36**) pp. 158–60, (**q42**) pp. 167–8, (**q44**) pp. 158–60, (**q46**) pp. 177–81, (**q47**) pp. 179–80, (**q48**) pp. 198–200, (**q49**) pp. 203–6, (**q50**) pp. 219–20, (**q51**) pp. 193–5, (**q55**) pp. 185–7, (**q56**) pp. 202–4, (**q57, q58**) pp. 208–10, (**q59**) pp. 218–19, (**q60**) pp. 206–7.

3  Devlin TM. *Textbook of Biochemistry with Clinical Correlations*. 6th ed. New York: Wiley-Liss; 2006. (**q33**) pp. 1013–15, (**q37**) pp. 536–9, (**q38**) pp. 908–9, (**q43**) pp. 13–16, (**q45**) pp. 15–18.

4  Brownie AC, Kernohan JC. *Medical Biochemistry*. 2nd ed. Edinburgh: Churchill Livingstone; 2005. (**q35**) pp. 58–61, (**q39**) pp. 260–5, (**q40**) pp. 290–5, (**q41**) pp. 75–9.

5 Alberts B, Johnson A, Lewis J, *et al. Molecular Biology of the Cell*. 4th ed. New York: Garland Science; 2002. (**q52**) pp. 10–12.

6 Berg JM, Tymoczko JL, Stryer, L. *Biochemistry*. 5th ed. New York: WH Freeman; 2002. (**q53**) pp. 465–84, 498–501.

7 Rosenfeld PJ, Brown DM, Heier JS, *et al*. Ranibizumab for neovascular age-related macular degeneration. *New Engl J Med*. 2006; **355**(14): 1419–31 (**q54**).

8 Kaufman P, Alm A. *Adler's Physiology of the Eye – clinical application*. 10th ed. Philadelphia: Mosby; 2003. (**q60**) pp. 397–8.

# 4. Pathology FRCOphth answers

1 **A** Oil Red O is used to stain lipid. Alcian blue stains mucopolysaccharides and periodic acid-Schiff (PAS) stains mucin. Fungi can be picked up with Grocott's hexamine. Congo red stains amyloid, which is deposited in the corneal stroma in lattice dystrophy. Amyloid can also be picked up using polarised light, exhibiting apple-green birefringence. Other stromal corneal dystrophies with characteristic histological staining patterns are granular dystrophy (hyaline deposits in the stroma stain with Masson trichrome) and macular dystrophy (glycosaminoglycans stain with Prussian blue). Other stains used in ophthalmology are Perl's Prussian blue for iron and alizarin red for calcium.[1,2]
**Difficulty level: 3**

2 **D** Hyperplasia is an increase in the number of cells in an organ or tissue. It can be physiological or pathological. Hypertrophy is an increase in the size of cells (or number of organelles in these cells) in an organ or tissue. It can be caused by increased functional demand, such as muscle hypertrophy in athletes or specific hormonal stimulation, such as uterine hypertrophy during pregnancy.

Breast enlargement during pregnancy, exercise-induced muscle change and uterine growth during pregnancy are all examples of physiological hypertrophy. The autoantibody produced in Graves' disease stimulates TSH receptors and causes thyroid hyperplasia.[3,4]
**Difficulty level: 4**

3 **C** The main influences on thrombosis are those constituting Virkow's triad: endothelial injury, changes in blood flow (such as stasis or turbulence) and hypercoagulabitlity.

Hypercoagulability may be primary (genetic) or secondary (acquired). Factor V Leiden, antithrombin III and protein C deficiencies are all primary causes of a hypercoagulable state, with factor V gene mutations being the most common. Hyper*viscosity (such as in polycythaemia rubra vera) and not hyp*oviscosity predisposes a patient to thrombosis. Other secondary causes of hypercoagulability include lupus anticoagulant (which, despite its name, has a procoagulant effect in vivo) and malignancy.[4]

**Difficulty level: 2**

4 **B** Basal cell carcinoma is the commonest malignant eyelid tumour, and usually affects the elderly. Most basal cell carcinomas are slow growing, and although invasive do not metastasise.

There are a few rare disorders that predispose to the development of multiple basal cell carcinomas in young people, which include Gorlin-Goltz syndrome and xeroderma pigmentosum. Treacher Collins syndrome is associated with colobomas of the eyelids, microphthalmos and mandibular hypoplasia.

Hermansky-Pudlak and Chédiak-Higashi syndromes are associated with oculocutaneous albinism – the former is associated with platelet dysfunction whereas the latter is associated with leucocytic abnormalities resulting in a susceptibility to infections.[2]

**Difficulty level: 4**

5 **B** Macrophages are the major cellular component of chronic inflammation. They are derived from monocytes that have been induced by chemokines and other factors. Macrophages are phagocytic cells and also secrete numerous proteases, complement components, cytokines such as interleukin 1 and tumour necrosis factor (TNF), and reactive oxygen species. Some of these components may also cause the tissue damage seen in chronic inflammation.

Granulomatous inflammation is a specific type of chronic inflammation in which the mediating cells are activated macrophages with an epitheloid appearance such as in tuberculosis. Lymphocytes, mast cells and eosinophils also play a role in chronic inflammation.[4]

**Difficulty level: 5**

6 **D** Gaucher's disease is an autosomal recessive condition characterised by reduced levels of glucocerebrosidase. This enzyme works on a fatty

substance called glucocerebroside, which if not acted upon accumulates in the spleen, liver, kidneys, lungs and brain. The disease is caused by a mutation in a gene located on chromosome 1 and affects both males and females.

All other conditions mentioned have an association with amyloid. Amyloidosis may also be found in certain patients with multiple myeloma (primary amyloidosis) and in chronic inflammatory states such as in rheumatoid arthritis or bronchiectasis (secondary amyloidosis).[4]

**Difficulty level: 5**

7　**A**　Retinoblastoma is the most common primary ocular malignancy in childhood. It may be heritable (40% of cases) or non-heritable (60% of cases).

The genetics of heritable retinoblastoma are described by the Knudson 'two-hit' hypothesis. One allele of the *RB1* gene contains a mutation in all cells. When a further mutation occurs in the other allele (second hit) the cell becomes malignant. If the child has heritable retinoblastoma with healthy parents, the risk to siblings is 2%. If a parent is affected, the risk to siblings is 40%.

If a patient has a solitary, unilateral retinoblastoma with no family history, this is probably (but not definitely) non-heritable, so the risk to each sibling of having the disease is 1%.[2]

**Difficulty level: 3**

8　**C**　Drusen are accumulations of extracellular material located between the RPE and Bruch's membrane, and are commonly (but not exclusively) seen in age-related macular degeneration. They consist of numerous proteins and lipids, the exact source of which is unclear. Clinically they appear yellow and may be described as hard (discrete, round, and less than half the size of the width of a retinal vein) and soft drusen (these have indistinct margins and vary in size but are often larger or equal to a vein width in diameter). They stain positive with periodic acid-Schiff (PAS) stain.[2]

**Difficulty level: 2**

9　**C**　Choroidal melanomas consist of spindle A, spindle B and epithelioid cell types. Spindle cells are thin, elongated and organised in tight bundles, whereas epithelioid cells are larger. Epithelioid cells are associated with the poorest prognosis. Other macroscopic pathological features include orbital spread, collar studding and subretinal fluid accumulation.

Many retinoblastomas consist of undifferentiated tissue. However, Flexner-Wintersteiner rosettes (these have a central lumen), Homer-Wright rosettes (no central lumen) and fleurettes are histological features of differentiated retinoblastoma. Fleurettes are foci of tumour cells that exhibit photoreceptor differentiation.

Palisading of cells is seen in basal cell carcinoma.[2]

**Difficulty level: 4**

**10 A** *NF1* (neurofibromatosis type 1) along with *p53* (multiple tumours), *BRCA1* (breast and ovarian cancer) are tumour suppressor genes, i.e. those that normally limit cell division and whose action is inactivated in cancer.

Oncogenes are genes whose products are associated with malignant change. Proto-oncogenes are normal genes which usually affect growth and cell division but can be converted into oncogenes by viruses or changes that affect their expression. *Myc* is involved in the development of Burkitt lymphoma, *abl* in chronic myeloid and acute lymphoblastic leukaemia and *erb-B1* in squamous cell carcinoma of the lung.[4]

**Difficulty level: 5**

**11 A** Optic nerve gliomas typically affect children with 75% of all optic nerve gliomas found in children aged under 10 years old. They may be asymptomatic, cause slowly progressive visual loss or proptosis. Histologically, the majority of cells are spindle-shaped pilocytic astrocytes and glial filaments. Optic nerve gliomas are associated with neurofibromatosis type 1 (NF1); the proportion of patients with NF1 is unclear, with reports ranging from 10% to 70% in the literature.

Tuberous sclerosis is associated with fundal astrocytomas, von Hippel-Lindau syndrome with retinal haemangiomas and Sturge-Weber syndrome with episcleral haemangiomas.[2,5]

**Difficulty level: 3**

**12 C** The pathological basis of atherosclerosis is thought to be due to endothelial injury causing a chronic inflammatory response. This injury may be as a result of hyperlipidaemia, hypertension, smoking, altered blood flow and many other causes.

There is subsequently increased endothelial permeability, leucocyte and platelet adhesion, increased coagulation and release of factors such as platelet-derived growth factor which promote migration of smooth muscle cells from the media into the intima and their proliferation, all of which contribute to the formation of a plaque.

There is a decrease in the nitric oxide : acetylcholine ratio. This results in a paradoxical vasoconstriction through the action of acetylcholine on smooth muscle.[4]
**Difficulty level: 5**

**13 C** Lacrimal gland carcinomas can be divided histologically into different types: (i) adenoid cystic, (ii) pleomorphic adenocarcinoma, (iii) mucoepidermoid and (iv) squamous cell. They are rare tumours.

Histology of lacrimal adenoid cystic carcinoma shows clusters of basaloid cells with solid areas and cribriform areas, the latter having a characteristic Swiss-cheese appearance.[2]
**Difficulty level: 3**

**14 A** Retinal emboli most commonly originate from an atheromatous plaque at the carotid bifurcation. They may consist of cholesterol (Hollenhorst plaques), calcium or platelets. Cholesterol emboli rarely cause major occlusion of retinal vessels. Calcific emboli tend to cause more extensive pathology such as branch or central retinal artery occlusions. Fibrin-platelet emboli may cause transient ischaemic attacks (amaurosis fugax) and occasionally complete obstruction. Another source of emboli may be from bacteria from cardiac vegetations in infective endocarditis.[2]
**Difficulty level: 1**

**15 D** Type I hypersensitivity (anaphylactic) is mediated by immunoglobulin E (IgE) antibodies.

Type II hypersensitivity (cytotoxic) is mediated by antibodies to intrinsic or extrinsic antigens on the cell surface. It is seen in myasthenia gravis and ocular cicatricial pemphigoid (OCP).

In Type III (immune complex mediated) hypersensitivity, immune complexes form between nuclear antigens and IgG antibodies such as in systemic lupus erythematosus.

Type IV (cell mediated) hypersensitivity is mediated by T-cells and leads to granulomatous inflammation.[4]
**Difficulty level: 3**

**16 A** Apoptosis, also known as programmed cell death, allows the selective removal of certain cells without disruption to surrounding areas. The cell membrane integrity is maintained, lysosomes remain intact and there is no inflammatory response. Characteristic chromatin condensation and DNA fragmentation are seen. This is in contrast to necrosis, where groups

of cells die and cell membrane integrity is disrupted in an uncontrolled manner.[4]
**Difficulty level: 2**

**17  C**  Hypoxia causes loss of ATP production by mitochondria. This affects functioning of sodium and potassium pumps, causing sodium influx into the cell accompanied by water resulting in cell swelling. Low oxygen levels lead to increased anaerobic glycolysis and accumulation of lactic acid which reduces cellular pH. There is reduced protein synthesis due to detachment of ribosomes from the endoplasmic reticulum.[4]
**Difficulty level: 4**

**18  B**  If the graft recipient has previously been exposed to antigens in the graft, for example via a prior blood transfusion, circulating antibodies to antigens in the graft will have formed. Therefore on receipt of the graft, within minutes to 2 days, antibodies fix to antigens in the graft, leading to complement activation and infiltration of platelets and neutrophils.

Other stages of rejection include: accelerated rejection (2–5 days), acute rejection (7–21 days) and chronic rejection (more than 3 months). Intimal fibrosis occurs in chronic rejection.[4]
**Difficulty level: 2**

**19  B**  Avellino dystrophy shows features of lattice and granular dystrophies. Histologically both hyaline and amyloid deposits are present. A useful mnemonic for stains in stromal dystrophy is:

Marilyn Monroe Always Gets Her Men in LA City
Macular – Mucopolysaccharide – Alcian blue
Granular – Hyaline – Masson trichrome
Lattice – Amyloid – Congo red

Colloidal iron also stains mucopolysaccharide and Alizarin red stains calcium.[6]
**Difficulty level: 3**

**20  B**  Prussian blue stains iron deposits.
Fleischer rings are iron deposits seen in keratoconus; a Stocker line is seen at the advancing edge of a pterygium and Ferry line at the base of a trabeculectomy bleb. Vogt striae are fine deep stromal striae seen in keratoconus and are not related to iron deposition.[2]
**Difficulty level: 2**

**21 B** Histological features of background diabetic retinopathy include loss of pericytes, thickening of basement membranes, and microaneurysm formation. Other clinical features include hard exudates and dot haemorrhages. In more advanced retinopathy, intraretinal microvascular abnormalities (IRMAs), cotton wool spots and blot haemorrhages are seen.

Deposition of amyloid is not classically associated with diabetic retinopathy.[2]

**Difficulty level: 2**

**22 C** Touton giant cells are seen in juvenile xanthogranuloma. This is a rare idiopathic granulomatous condition due to proliferation of non-Langerhans histiocytes. Cutaneous yellow papules and yellow lesions on the iris are seen.

Giant cell arteritis is characterised by a fragmented internal elastic lamina, giant cells, leucocyte infiltration and intimal fibrosis.

In tuberculosis, there is a granulomatous inflammatory response with epithelioid cells, occasional Langhans giant cells, lymphocytes and fibroblasts. Caseating necrosis of the granulomas may be seen. In sarcoidosis, non-caseating granulomas form in which Langhans and foreign body giant cells are seen.[2,4]

**Difficulty level: 3**

**23 C** This is a corneal endothelial dystrophy. Initial features are of corneal guttata (excrescences of Descemet's membrane rather than Bowman's) and in more advanced cases the endothelium taken on a beaten-bronze appearance.

Endothelial decompensation may ensue leading to blurred vision and stromal oedema. In advanced cases there is epithelial oedema and microcysts and bullous keratopathy may develop.[2]

**Difficulty level: 2**

**24 B** The difference between benign and malignant tumours is based on their (i) differentiation, (ii) rate of growth, (iii) local invasion and (iv) ability to metastasise. Benign tumours tend to be well differentiated, whereas malignant tumours tend to be poorly differentiated, showing nuclear and cellular pleomorphism and many nuclear mitoses. Malignant tumours also tend to grow more rapidly, be locally invasive and most have the ability to metastasise.[4]

**Difficulty level: 2**

**25 C** Epstein-Barr virus is associated with Burkitt's lymphoma and nasopharyngeal carcinoma. Hepatitis B virus and also hepatitis C virus are associated with hepatocellular carcinoma, possibly due to the chronic infective state associated with them. Hepatitis A usually causes a self-limiting infection with no chronic component. Human immunodeficiency virus is associated with lymphoma and predisposes to many other types of tumour; for example, Kaposi sarcoma.[4]
**Difficulty level: 2**

**26 D** Shock is a state of reduced systemic perfusion due to decreased cardiac output or circulating blood volume. Major classes are hypovolaemic, cardiogenic, septic and anaphylactic.

Seventy per cent of septic shock is caused by Gram-negative bacilli expressing endotoxin (consisting of bacterial lipopolysaccharides released with the degradation of bacterial cell walls).[4]
**Difficulty level: 3**

**27 C** Most surgical wounds heal via primary intention: the edges of the wound are opposed using sutures, staples or tape and the incision space is filled initially by clot and then by granulation tissue and collagen. Healing is faster.

Secondary intention is used for large wounds whose edges are difficult to oppose. They are not sutured and granulation tissue grows in from the margins to fill the defect. The wound also contracts due to the presence of myofibroblasts. Healing is slower and more likely to leave a larger scar.[4]
**Difficulty level: 2**

**28 D** Hyperplasia occurs when there is an increase in cell number by mitosis. Hypertrophy is seen when there is an increase in cell size without cell division. Metaplasia is the reversible transformation of one differentiated cell type into another differentiated cell type. Dysplasia is seen when there is increased cell growth with atypia and decreased differentiation.[3]
**Difficulty level: 2**

**29 C** In angiogenesis, new blood vessels grow from pre-existing blood vessels. This is controlled partly by growth factors and receptors, such as vascular endothelial growth factor (VEGF) and platelet derived growth factor (PDGF). VEGF inhibition is now used commonly in the treatment of neovascular age-related macular degeneration.

Other regulatory factors in angiogenesis are extracellular matrix proteins such as integrins and matrix metalloproteases. There are also

inhibitors of angiogenesis such as interferon-alpha and thrombospondin. Serotonin is not known to be involved in the process of angiogenesis.[4]
**Difficulty level: 4**

**30 C** Histological features of common skin cancers are:
- basal cell carcinoma – palisading of cells
- squamous cell carcinoma – keratin pearls
- cutaneous melanoma – pigmented spindle-shaped cells
- sebaceous cell carcinoma – foamy cytoplasm and pagetoid spread.[2]
**Difficulty level: 3**

# References

1 Yanoff M, Sassani JW. *Ocular Pathology*. 6th ed. Maryland Heights: Mosby, Elsevier; 2009. (**q1**) p. 1058.
2 Kanski JJ. *Clinical Ophthalmology – a systematic approach*. 6th ed. Edinburgh: Butterworth Heinemann Elsevier; 2007. (**q1**) pp. 295–8, (**q4**) pp. 109–10, (**q7**) pp. 543–5, (**q8**) p. 629–31, (**q9**) pp. 110, 530–1, 542–4, (**q11**) pp. 195–8, 917–21, (**q13**) pp. 193–5, (**q14**) p. 593, (**q20**) pp. 243, 288, (**q21**) pp. 567, 575, (**q22**) p. 522, (**q23**) p. 300, (**q30**) pp. 110–15.
3 Underwood JCE, Cross SS. *General and Systematic Pathology*, 5th ed. Edinburgh: Churchill Livingstone Elsevier; 2009. (**q2, q28**) pp. 78–9, (**q28**) pp. 82–3.
4 Kumar V, Abbas AK, Fausto N, *et al. Robbins and Cotran Pathologic Basis of Disease*. 8th ed. Philadelphia: Saunders Elsevier; 2010. (**q2**) pp. 6–8, (**q3**) pp. 121–2, (**q5**) p. 71, (**q6**) pp. 251–3, (**q10**) pp. 281, 287, (**q12**) pp. 496–502, (**q15**) pp. 198–205, (**q16**) pp. 14–26, (**q17**) pp. 23–4, (**q18**) pp. 226–30, (**q22**) pp. 73, 371, 512–13, (**q24**) pp. 262–9, (**q25**) pp. 314–15, (**q26**) pp. 129–32, (**q27**) p. 102, (**q29**) pp. 100–1.
5 Wilhelm H. Primary optic nerve tumours. *Curr Opin Neurol*. 2009; **22**(1): 11–18 (**q11**).
6 Wong TW. *The Ophthalmological Examinations Review*. Singapore: World Scientific Publishing; 2007. (**q19**) p. 112.

# 4. Pathology ICO answers

**31**   i.  F       ii.  F       iii.  T       iv.  F       v.  F

Intracranial meningioma can commonly cause a rise in intracranial pressure, with resultant papilloedema. Only meningiomas that arise from the olfactory groove or the sphenoid commonly result in optic atrophy. Furthermore, they can also cause a 6th nerve palsy which is described as a false localising sign. Pathologically, psammoma bodies are visible. Meningiomas are the most commonly detected primary intracranial neoplasms, accounting for 25% of all lesions detected in the United States. Most cases are sporadic, but some can be familial. Recent frequent genetic mutations involved in meningiomas are inactivation mutations in the *NF2* gene (merlin) on chromosome 22q. The *MN1* gene is also thought to play a role in some cases and is also located on chromosome 22q.[1,2]
**Difficulty level: 3**

**32**   i.  F       ii.  F       iii.  T       iv.  T       v.  F

Inflammatory cells are often present in the media and intima, the latter of which may often be fragmented. Tongue claudication is a pathognomonic sign, and in between 5% to 10% of cases, the patient may have a normal ESR and CRP. Giant cell arteritis is commonly linked with polymyalgia rheumatica (PMR). It is more common in females than males in the ratio 3 : 1, and it is extremely rare in those aged below 50. Recent advances in MRI imaging using high resolution and contrast injection have suggested that this condition can now be detected and diagnosed non-invasively, with high specificity and sensitivity.[1,3,4]
**Difficulty level: 3**

**33**   i.  T       ii.  F       iii.  F       iv.  F       v.  F

Pterygia are thought to occur through environmental exposure to wind and ultraviolet light, although recent case reports highlighting pterygia in children and twins lends support to a potential genetic predilection. Basophils predominate on section, along with the absence of cystic spaces and stromal elastosis. Fibroblastic proliferation is also present commonly. Sometimes a line of iron can be seen at the head of the pterygium known as Stocker's line, with Fuchs'

patches (grey blemishes that disperse around the pterygium head) also visible. Conjunctival autografts and the use of topical mitomycin C have established favourable outcomes in recent years.[5-7]
**Difficulty level: 4**

**34**    i. T      ii. F      iii. T      iv. T      v. F

Periodic acid-Schiff (PAS) only stains some viruses. It is mainly used to stain structures containing a high proportion of carbohydrate macromolecules. It can also be used to differentiate between different types of glycogen storage diseases. *Acanthamoeba* cysts can be picked up using PAS (stains purple), Grocott's hexamine (stains black) and green fluorescence is seen with calcofluor white. Haemotoxylin and eosin stains involve the application of haemalum, which is a complex formed of aluminium ions and oxidized haematoxylin. This colours nuclei of cells blue. The nuclear staining is followed by counterstaining with an aqueous or alcoholic solution of eosin Y, which colours eosinophilic structures a shade of red, pink and orange.[6]
**Difficulty level: 4**

**35**    i. T      ii. T      iii. F      iv. T      v. F

Interleukin 8 is a potent neutrophil chemoattractant and is secreted by activated macrophages and other cell types. It has limited activity on eosinophils and monocytes. Interleukin 7 is a potent haematopoietic growth factor that is secreted by stromal cells in the marrow and thymus. Wound healing by primary intention does not involve a breach of the dermis. The proliferation phase is initiated by growth factors FGF, EGF, PDGF and TNF and occurs later in the wound-healing process (after day 7). Degradation of collagen is completed by metalloproteinases, which are essential in the wound-healing process. These act on fibronectin, laminin and other extracellular matrix components for remodelling.[1,8]
**Difficulty level: 4**

**36**    i. T      ii. F      iii. T      iv. F      v. F

Colloidal iron stains mucopolysaccharides blue and is useful in the diagnosis of macular corneal dystrophy, which is inherited in an autosomal recessive fashion and is thought to result in an abnormal configuration of keratin sulphate. The iron particles are stabilised in ammonia and glycerine and are attracted to acid mucopolysaccharides. Iron can be identified using Perl's Prussian blue. Alcian blue is useful in the detection of mucopolysaccharides in macular corneal dystrophy. Congo red is useful in the detection of amyloid, which can often be present in post-mortems of patients with Alzheimer's disease. Specimens can also exhibit apple-green birefringence with polarised light.[6]

**Difficulty level: 4**

**37**  i. T  ii. F  iii. T  iv. T  v. T

Hypertrophy occurs in cardiac or skeletal muscle in response to exercise, and also in the liver. It involves an increase in both cell size but not cell number. The increase in cell size is due to an increase in synthesis of structural components. This increase can be due to an increase in functional demand or due to hormonal stimulation. In the heart, the most common stimulus is haemodynamic overload. The phenotype of cells can also be changed by hypertrophy. In cardiac muscle during volume overload, there is a switch of contractile proteins to foetal forms with alterations resulting in slower velocity of contraction in the hypertrophied fibres.[1,8]

**Difficulty level: 1**

**38**  i. T  ii. F  iii. T  iv. F  v. F

Macular corneal dystrophy occurs as a consequence of a systemic error in keratan sulphate metabolism. Inheritance is autosomal recessive with gene locus on 16q21. There are three subgroups, depending on the degree of presence of antigenic keratan sulphate. Abnormal aggregations of glycosaminoglycans stain with Alcian blue, and histologically the collagen is closely packed. The pH of Alcian blue can be adjusted to increase specificity. Clinically, the condition is characterised by multiple grey-white opacities that are present in the corneal stroma and extend into the peripheral cornea. The changes usually become visible in the first decade of life and a reduction in acuity can occur by the age of 40. Surgical treatment can include full or partial thickness corneal grafting.[6]

**Difficulty level: 4**

**39**  i. T  ii. T  iii. F  iv. T  v. F

Metastases can spread through the lymphatic system and tumours of this type express a number of molecules on their cell surfaces. The pattern of lymph node dissemination follows natural routes of drainage. Local lymph nodes can sometimes be bypassed, so-called skip metastases, due to venous-lymphatic anastomoses, or due to other causes such as inflammation or radiation. Due to the increase in growth rate cell membranes increase glucose transport. The liver is the most common site for metastases. In bone metastases, an increase in both osteoclastic and osteoblastic activity is observed. Metastatic cells often express numerous motility factors, as well as adhesion receptors.[1]

**Difficulty level: 4**

---

**40**   i. F      ii. T      iii. T      iv. T      v. T

Choroidal melanomas contain spindle A, B and epitheloid cell types. A collar stud appearance is evident, often on B-scan ultrasonography. Spindle A cells contain slender nuclei with absent chromatin and no mitotic activity. The cytoplasm can sometimes contain melanin granules. Spindle B cells contain plump nuclei with small nucleoli and coarse chromatin. Mitotic figures are common. Epithelioid predominant choroidal melanomas carry the worst prognosis, with approximately 35% survival at 15 years. Lesions composed of spindle cells are less aggressive and do not tend to metastasise. The survival of this latter group is approximately 75% at 15 years. Clinical treatment can include careful monitoring, radiation therapy or enucleation.[1]

**Difficulty level: 4**

---

**41**   i. T      ii. T      iii. F      iv. F      v. T

Vascular permeability leads to the release of protein-rich exudate into the extravascular space. As protein-rich fluid is lost from the blood vessel, the extravascular oncotic pressure increases. The normal hydrostatic pressure of a capillary at its arterial end is about 32 mmHg, and at its venous end approximately 12 mmHg. Together with an increase in hydrostatic pressure the net result is vascular leakage. This is a hallmark of acute inflammation. A variety of mechanisms can induce vascular leakage, notably endothelial contraction, direct injury, a regenerating endothelium and leucocyte-dependent leakage.[1]

**Difficulty level: 3**

---

**42**   i. T      ii. T      iii. F      iv. F      v. T

Metaplasia is a reversible phenomenon in which an adult cell type is replaced by another cell type. The most common adaptive metaplasia is squamous cell metaplasia in the human lung, and this occurs in the lungs in response to chronic irritation, for example by cigarette smoke. Another example of metaplasia is in Barrett's oesophagus, where the squamous oesophageal epithelium is replaced by gastric columnar cells. It is a deficiency of vitamin A (retinoic acid) that can induce a squamous metaplasia in the respiratory epithelium.

Metaplasia may occur in mesenchymal cells, and the very control of cell differentiation, using growth factors and other chemicals is of great interest with stem cell research.[1]

**Difficulty level: 3**

**43**   **i.** F      **ii.** T      **iii.** F      **iv.** T      **v.** T

During cell injury, nuclear changes can appear in three characteristic patterns. Karyolysis implies the fading of nuclear chromatin and the term karyorrhexis implies nuclear fragmentation. Once the necrotic cells have undergone early changes gross morphological characteristics may be observed. Coagulative necrosis is often visible in myocardial infarction, in which the necrotic myocardial cells are removed by fragmentation and phagocytosis of the cellular debris by scavenger cells. Caseous necrosis is often present in tuberculosis infection, and enzymatic fat necrosis can occur in the pancreas.[1]

**Difficulty level: 4**

**44**   **i.** T      **ii.** T      **iii.** F      **iv.** F      **v.** T

A large case series of 311 patients with primary acquired melanosis (PAM) was analysed retrospectively by Shields *et al.* in 2007. They found that in those with histological confirmation of PAM without atypia, none progressed to melanoma, whereas 13% of the PAM with atypia group did. Other case series have suggested an even higher proportion of the latter group progress to melanoma, with those with a pagetoid growth pattern having the worst prognosis. The size and extent of PAM with atypia correlated with the risk of progression to melanoma, with 6 clock hours of PAM having a 6.8 times relative increase in risk compared to PAM of 1 clock hour. Conjunctival melanomas often present in the fifth to sixth decade of life, but rarely arise de novo. Approximately 20% arise from pre-existing naevi, and 75% from PAM with atypia.[9]

**Difficulty level: 4**

**45**   **i.** T      **ii.** T      **iii.** F      **iv.** F      **v.** F

Cytoplasmic c-ANCA, an antineutrophil anticytoplasmic antibody is present in the majority of patients with Wegener's granulomatosis. Perinuclear p-ANCA is directed towards myeloperoxidase, and is far more common in polyarteritis nodosa (PAN). The presence and concentration of ANCA titres correlates well with disease severity. So far, no antibodies have been detected in giant cell arteritis, whereas antiendothelial antibodies are present in Kawasaki's syndrome. Antibodies to DNA complexes have been observed in systemic lupus erythematosus (SLE). Syphilis is a spirochetal infection and can induce an infectious vaculitis, along with Herpesviridae and bacteria such as *Neisseria*.[1]

**Difficulty level: 4**

**46**   i.  F       ii.  F       iii.  T       iv.  T       v.  F

Lattice corneal dystrophy is an autosomal dominant disorder characterised by fine lines criss-crossing the stroma. Macular dystrophy is autosomal recessive whereas granular dystrophy is autosomal dominant. Opaque 'granules' within the transparent tissue are features of the anterior corneal stroma, along with staining of a keratin-like substance, known as keratinoid. Labrador keratopathy consists of the deposition of golden-yellow particles of protein beneath the epithelium, in the superficial stroma and Bowman's layer. It often occurs in patients with chronic or excessive sunlight exposure. Fuchs' endothelial dystrophy consists of thickening of Descemet's membrane with loss of endothelial cell number. Excrescences of Descemet's are known as Hassall-Henle bodies.[10]

**Difficulty level: 4**

**47**   i.  T       ii.  T       iii.  T       iv.  T       v.  F

Diabetic eye disease is a leading cause of blindness, and if unmonitored can lead to sight-threatening complications. The retinal circulation undergoes change and the presence of new blood vessels, either at the disc or elsewhere, are features of proliferative diabetic retinopathy. Cranial nerve palsies can affect the extraocular muscles, such as a 6th cranial nerve causing lateral rectus palsy and thereby inducing diplopia. Diabetic patients are more prone to posterior subcapsular cataracts and have poorly healing epithelia. Diabetic maculopathy is treatable with laser or intravitreal steroid, and new research is focusing upon anti-VEGF treatments that are likely to have a role in the future.[10]

**Difficulty level: 2**

**48**    i. F         ii. T         iii. T         iv. T         v. T

Homocystinuria is characterised by a reduction in cystathione β-synthetase levels, which increases the potential risk of thrombus formation. Inferonasal lens dislocation is a pathognomonic feature of homocystinuria, and histological examination of this reveals PAS-positive material. Cystinosis is characterised by the deposition of crystals on the cornea, conjunctiva, choroid and retina. The biochemical abnormality occurs in the continual release of cystine within the lysosomes and its inefficient release. One to two per cent of renal stones can be due to cystine. Other systemic features of cystinosis can include growth retardation, hepatosplenomegaly and hypothyroidism.[6,10]

**Difficulty level: 4**


**49**    i. T         ii. T         iii. F         iv. T         v. F

Neurofibromatosis is an autosomal dominant condition characterised by an overgrowth of neural supportive tissue. Lisch nodules consist of melanocytic proliferations of the iris, and goniodysgenesis may also occur. Retinal glial tumours and optic nerve glioma are other features. In tuberous sclerosis, small yellow tumours form within the retina known as astrocytic hamartomas. Elsewhere, tumours may be detected in the walls of the cerebral ventricles, with angiomyolipomas detected in the renal cortex and rhabdomyomas located in the myocardium.

Sturge-Weber syndrome is not inherited, and consists of vascular malformations over the facial skin. Glaucoma can occur due to an impairment of aqueous outflow, principally due to proliferation of vascular tissue in the anterior chamber drainage angle, as well as episcleral vascular malformations causing increased resistance.[10]

**Difficulty level: 2**


**50**    i. F         ii. T         iii. T         iv. T         v. T

Flow cytometry is a technique used to identify phenotypically different cells from a larger, mixed population. It uses the principle of staining specific antigens on cell surfaces using fluorescein labelled antibodies. Cells are passed through a fluorescence activated cell sorter (FACS). Avidin biotin is useful for paraffin section analysis, and Ki67 is a nuclear protein which maintains DNA during mitosis. Ki67 antibodies are thus used and allow the detection of the rate of proliferation. Impression cytology is useful; for example, in vitamin A deficiency where there is a loss of goblet cells and surface keratinisation occurs. Haematoxylin and eosin are the most commonly used stains in histopathology.[10]

**Difficulty level: 3**

**51**  i. F  ii. T  iii. F  iv. T  v. F

Exophthalmos due to thyroid eye disease may be unilateral or bilateral. Hyperthyroidism is usually associated with elevated serum $T_3$ and $T_4$ levels, with a reciprocal decrease in thyroid stimulating hormone levels. On magnetic resonance imaging (MRI) there is often uniform swelling of extraocular muscles, and the tendons are spared. On histological analysis of extraocular muscle, a perivascular infiltration of lymphocytes is visible, and if left untreated the muscles eventually fibrose. Larger axons of the motor nerves supplying the muscles are reduced, resulting in a limitation of eye movement and subsequent ophthalmoplegia. Clinically, patients with thyroid eye disease can present with ocular surface symptoms due to lagophthlmos and proptosis, along with diplopia from muscle restriction.[10]

**Difficulty level: 2**

**52**  i. F  ii. T  iii. F  iv. F  v. F

Dot haemorrhages typically represent capillary haemorrhage into the outer plexiform layer, whereas flame haemorrhages tend to be larger and arrow-like, tracking in the nerve fibre layer. Blot haemorrhages are round and large, often tracking between the retinal pigment epithelium and photoreceptor layer. Intraretinal microvascular abnormalities, or IRMAs, are commonly seen in poorly controlled diabetics and consist of irregular segmental growth and dilatation of blood vessels from the venous side of the circulation into an area of retinal hypoperfusion. These areas often leak on fundus fluorescein angiography. Retinopathy of prematurity is characterised by abnormal proliferation of new blood vessels stimulated by a return to normal ambient oxygen levels. These vessels can rupture and bleed into the vitreous.[10]

**Difficulty level: 3**

**53**  i. T  ii. F  iii. T  iv. F  v. T

Reversible cell injury is characterised by mitochondrial swelling in response to hypoxia. Glycogen stores are rapidly depleted as the cell switches to anaerobic metabolism. Early clumping of chromatin occurs, along with bleb formation of the cell membrane. As the cell swells due to solute accumulation, swelling of the endoplasmic reticulum also occurs, along with autophagy of lysosomes. Up to a point, if normal oxygenation is restored, these changes are reversible. In contrast, irreversible cell injury is characterised by nuclear pyknosis and karyolysis, along with endoplasmic reticulum lysis. Lysosomal lysis also occurs, and defects are found within the cell membrane.[1]

**Difficulty level: 3**

**54**  i. F      ii. T      iii. T      iv. T      v. F

Vasoconstriction in inflammation is often induced by thromboxane $A_2$, along with leukotrienes $C_4$ and $D_4$. Thromboxane $A_2$ is also a potent platelet aggregator. Leukotriene $B_4$ induces chemotaxis, and platelet activating factor is derived from mast cells, neutrophils, platelets and endothelium. It is a phospholipid-derived mediator and has major inflammatory actions, including decreased vascular permeability, leucocyte aggregation and adhesion, platelet activation and the stimulation of other mediators including leukotrienes and interleukins. These secondary effects increase leucocyte integrin binding to cells, mast cell degranulation and the oxidative burst. In experimental models, PAF antagonists inhibit inflammation.[1]

**Difficulty level: 3**

**55**  i. T      ii. T      iii. T      iv. T      v. T

Interleukin 1, along with tumour necrosis factor alpha (TNF-$\alpha$) affects the thermoregulatory centre of the brain to induce a state of fever. They are produced from activated macrophages and their production can be stimulated by immune complexes, bacterial endotoxins or direct injury. Interleukin 1 has autocrine, paracrine and endocrine effects. It has secondary affects of reducing appetite and inducing neutrophilia. Effects on the endothelium can include leucocyte adherence, prostaglandin synthesis, an increase in procoagulant activity and an increase in production of other interleukins. Other effects of interleukin 1 include an increase in collagen synthesis, proliferation, and protease release. There is an increase in prostaglandin synthesis.[1]

**Difficulty level: 2**

**56**  i. T      ii. T      iii. T      iv. T      v. T

Fibroblast growth factor (FGF) plays a pivotal role in the wound-healing process, helping to remodel connective tissue and parenchymal constituents following the acute inflammatory process, along with collagenisation and acquisition of wound strength. FGF is pivotal in monocyte chemotaxis, fibroblast migration, fibroblast proliferation, angiogenesis and collagenase secretion. Collagen synthesis itself is induced by tumour growth factor β, platelet-derived growth factor, and tumour necrosis factor α. It is thought that FGF plays a role in the production of matrix metalloproteinases (MMPs), gelatinases and stromelysins, which help to degrade collagen and remodel the healing tissue.[1]

**Difficulty level: 2**

**57**   **i.** T      **ii.** T      **iii.** F      **iv.** T      **v.** F

Basal cell carcinoma is often present on the upper or lower eyelids and may manifest as an ulcer with rolled or poorly defined edges. The most common types are solid basal cell carcinomas with prominent mitotic figures, and in the periphery, the cells are arranged in palisades. Basal cell carcinomas occur in Gorlin-Goltz syndrome. Other malignancies in this syndrome can include medulloblastoma, breast carcinoma and Hodgkin's lymphoma. Morphoeic basal cell carcinomas induce a marked fibroblastic response which overshadows the proliferating basal cells. Sclerosing basal cell carcinomas do not have a distinct border and a wide excision is often required.[1]

**Difficulty level: 4**

**58**   **i.** F      **ii.** T      **iii.** F      **iv.** T      **v.** F

Conjunctival melanomas carry a 10% mortality rate at 5 years, and this increases to 25% at 10 years. Whilst commonly developing on the bulbar conjunctiva, they can present anywhere and placement in the fornix, caruncle or palpebral conjunctiva carries a poorer prognosis. Common sites for metastases include the brain, lung and cervical regional lymph nodes. Topical mitomycin C has been used to control local tumour recurrence with some effect (Damato *et al.*). Amelanotic melanomas are unusually a fleshy pink colour. Conjunctival melanomas typically arise from primary acquired melanosis (PAM) in 75% of cases, with approximately 20% of cases arising from conjunctival naevi and 2%–3% cases arising de novo.[6,11]

**Difficulty level: 4**

**59**   **i.** F      **ii.** F      **iii.** F      **iv.** F      **v.** T

Grocott's hexamine silver is used to stain fungi, although it also stains glycogen, mucins, amoebae and melanin as well. Gram staining is commonly performed in histology, and the method involves first staining with crystal violet blue-black, then iodine, followed by decolourising with acetone. After this, counterstaining with carbol-fuschin is performed. Acridine orange may also be used for fungi, whereas Ziehl–Neelsen staining is conducted to detect *Mycobacterium tuberculosis*. Giemsa staining methods are used to detect chlamydial elements. Hansel's stain, eosin-methylene blue mixture, is used for the rapid detection of eosinophils.[10]

**Difficulty level: 3**

**60**  i. T  ii. F  iii. F  iv. T  v. F

Sarcoidosis is characterised by a non-caseating granulomatous inflammatory process, and can affect a number of visceral organs as well as the skin. It frequently causes an increase in vitamin D production outside the kidney. A Kveim test is valuable to confirm the diagnosis, but is rarely used in clinical practice. Serum angiotensin converting enzyme (ACE) is useful but is generally less specific. Within the eye, sarcoidosis can induce conjunctiva and uveal tract inflammation, and can present on the iris and ciliary body as nodules (Boeck's sarcoid). Lisch nodules are usually found on this iris in neurofibromatosis. Similarly, as a solid mass, sarcoid can deposit around the eye and lacrimal gland. Histologically, macrophages form multinucleate giant cells and palisades of epithelial like cells around a focus of tissue destruction.[10]

**Difficulty level: 4**

## References

1  Kumar V, Abbas AK, Fausto N, *et al. Robbins and Cotran Pathologic Basis of Disease.* 7th ed. Philadelphia: Saunders Elsevier; 2005. (**q31**) pp. 1349–51, (**q32**) pp. 694–5, (**q35**) pp. 71, 84–5, (**q37**) pp. 44–6, (**q39**) pp. 250–1, (**q40**) pp. 1181–2, (**q41**) pp. 54–6, (**q42**) pp. 48–9, (**q43**) pp. 16–17, (**q45**) pp. 490–1, (**q53**) pp. 6–7, (**q54, q55**) pp. 70–1, (**q56**) pp. 88–9, (**q57**) pp. 1187–8.

2  Kwagoe H, Grosveld GC. MN1-TEL myeloid oncoprotein expressed in multipotent progenitors perturbs both myeloid and lymphoid growth and causes T-lymphoid tumors in mice. *Blood.* 2005; **106**(13): 4278–86 (**q31**).

3  Hayreh SS. Risk factors in AION. *Ophthalmology.* 2001; **108**(10): 1717–18 (**q32**).

4  Bley TA, Uhl M, Carew J, *et al.* Diagnostic value of high-resolution MR imaging in giant cell arteritis. *Am J Neuroradiol.* 2007; **28**(9): 1722–7 (**q32**).

5  Trikha S, Khan-Lim D, Evans A. Successful surgical intervention of a childhood pterygium using a conjunctival autograft. *J Paediatr Ophthalmol Strabismus.* 2010; **2**: 1–3 (**q33**).

6 Kanski JJ. *Clinical Ophthalmology – a systematic approach*. 6th ed. Edinburgh: Butterworth Heinemann Elsevier; 2007. (**q33**) p. 84, (**q34**) pp. 105–6, (**q36**) p. 1328, (**q38**) pp. 128–9, (**q48**) p. 138, (**q58**) pp. 88–9.

7 Coroneo MT. Pterygium as an early indicator of ultraviolet insolation: a hypothesis. *Br J Ophthalmol*. 1993; **77**(11): 734–9 (**q33**).

8 Guyton A, Hall J. *Textbook of Medical Physiology*. 10th ed. Philadelphia: Saunders; 2001. (**q35**) p. 143, (**q37**) p. 13.

9 Shields JA, Shields CL, Mashayeki A, *et al*. Primary acquired melanosis of the conjunctiva: experience with 311 cases. *Trans Am Exp Ophthalmol*. 2007; **105**: 65–72 (**q44**).

10 Forrester J, Dick A, McMenamin A, *et al*. The Eye: basic sciences in practice. 2nd ed. Philadelphia: Saunders Elsevier; 2007. (**q46**) pp. 407–8, (**q47**) pp. 404–5, (**q48**) p. 405, (**q49**) pp. 414–15, (**q50**) pp. 432–3, (**q51**) p. 404, (**q52**) p. 402, (**q59**) pp. 7–8, (**q60**) pp. 388–9.

11 Demirci H, McCormick SA, Finger PT. Topical mitomycin C chemotherapy for conjunctival malignant melanoma and primary acquired melanosis with atypia. *Arch Ophthalmol*. 2000; **118**: 885–91 (**q58**).

# 5. Microbiology and immunology FRCOphth answers

**1** **D** Fungi such as *Candida* species and parasites are eukaryotic. Bacteria, *Rickettsia* and *Chlamydia* are prokaryotes. *Rickettsia* and *Chlamydia* are Gram-negative organisms; bacteria may be Gram negative or Gram positive.[1]
**Difficulty level: 2**

**2** **C** In order to cause damage, bacteria need to adhere to and invade host cells as well as delivering toxic components. Genes encoding virulence properties are sometimes physically associated and are called pathogenicity islands. Structures such as fibrillae, fimbriae or pili allow adherence to host cells. Mycobacteria are able to inhibit the host cell's normal protective mechanism of lysosomal digestion. Endotoxins are lipopolysaccharide components of Gram-negative bacterial cell walls.[2]
**Difficulty level: 3**

3   **C**   Staphylococci are Gram-positive cocci, Clostridia are Gram-positive bacilli, *Neisseria* are Gram-negative cocci and *Pseudomonas* are Gram-negative bacilli. The bacterial cell wall, as well as determining Gram staining, also affects antibiotic penetration and action.[3]
    **Difficulty level: 3**

4   **B**   Other commensals include other *Neisseria* species, *Staphylococcus epidermidis* and *Staphylococcus aureus*. Answers a, c and d may cause bacterial conjunctivitis.[4]
    **Difficulty level: 2**

5   **D**   Viruses may be classified according to the DNA or RNA component of their core. Herpes viruses such as herpes simplex, cytomegalovirus and Epstein-Barr virus are DNA viruses. Adenovirus is also a DNA virus. RNA viruses include paramyxoviruses such as measles and retroviruses such as HIV.[7]
    **Difficulty level: 4**

6   **A**   Aciclovir is converted to the triphosphate form in infected cells and inhibits viral DNA polymerase. It is particularly effective against herpes simplex and varicella zoster viruses. It has only a small effect on cytomegalovirus, which is better treated with ganciclovir or foscarnet. Aciclovir triphosphate is quickly broken down by host cells, and may cause renal dysfunction with intravenous use.[3]
    **Difficulty level: 3**

7   **D**   HIV is an RNA retrovirus, most commonly detected by serology using ELISA or Western blots. The WHO staging system states AIDS is only diagnosed when the patient develops a specified AIDS-defining illness. However, the Centers for Disease Control (CDC) guidelines consider any HIV-positive person with a CD4 count under 200 to have AIDS. The development of Kaposi sarcoma is associated with HHV-8 infection in HIV patients.[2]
    **Difficulty level: 3**

8   **B**   Vertical transmission of syphilis is a risk factor for the development of interstitial keratitis. Trauma, diabetes, immunosuppression, chronic ocular surface disease and use of hydrophilic contact lenses are risk factors for fungal keratitis.[5]
    **Difficulty level: 3**

**9  B**  *Acanthamoeba* is a free-living protozoan, and may cause keratitis, commonly associated with contact lens wear. It can be stained with periodic acid-Schiff (PAS) or calcofluor white, and is cultured on non-nutrient agar seeded with dead *E. coli*. Treatment is with debridement and topical amoebicides (propamidine isethionate and polyhexamethylene biguanide drops or hexamidine and chlorhexidine).[5]
**Difficulty level: 3**

**10  B**  Sterilisation involves the destruction of bacteria and their spores (as opposed to disinfection which involves destruction of the microorganisms only). It uses exposure to moist heat at 121°C for 15 minutes. It can be used to sterilise porous materials such as theatre clothing, paper packs, rubber and solution-containing bottles. Commercially, ionizing radiation is used to sterilise prepacked disposable instruments such as plastic syringes.[4]
**Difficulty level: 2**

**11  A**  Aminoglycosides are effective against many aerobic Gram-negative and some Gram-positive organisms. They act via inhibiting bacterial protein synthesis and are bactericidal. They do not penetrate the blood-brain barrier and so do not enter the vitreous. They are metabolised by the kidney and may cause nephrotoxicity, especially in patients with pre-existing renal disease, or if other nephrotoxic agents are used.[3]
**Difficulty level: 3**

**12  A**  Ciprofloxacin is a fluoroquinolone antibiotic and acts via inhibition of DNA gyrase. It has a broad spectrum of action and is effective in treating Gram-positive and Gram-negative bacteria. Ciprofloxacin has good ocular penetration. It has no cross-reactivity with patients sensitive to cephalosporins (it is in patients with penicillin sensitivity that there is 10% cross-reactivity with cephalosporins).[3]
**Difficulty level: 3**

**13  C**  The constituents of the innate immune system are not affected by previous contact with the infectious agent. They include external barriers against infection such as the integrity of skin or mucosa, which can be aided by secretions that are toxic to pathogens such as lysozyme in tears. Phagocytes, complement, acute phase proteins and natural killer cells are also parts of the innate immune system. Cytotoxic T-cells are part of specific acquired immunity.[6]
**Difficulty level: 3**

**14 C** Immunoglobulins are Y-shaped molecules and consist of two light chains and two heavy chains. The arms of the Y are named the Fab region and stem the Fc region. The Fab region binds to antigen and the Fc region determines immunoglobulin class.

Each constituent chain contains a variable (V) and constant (C) region. Heavy chains also have a diversity (D) region.

Antibody diversity is generated by recombination events of the multiple gene segments in the heavy and light chain gene loci. The heavy chain variable region is determined by rearrangement of the V, D and J encoding gene loci (the C region remains constant). The light chain gene is constructed by joining of V and J genes.[6]

**Difficulty level: 4**

**15 C** MALT is a collection of subepithelial antigen presenting cells and lymphoid tissue and is not contained within a capsule. It is present on mucosal surfaces including the conjunctiva and ocular adnexal glands. The predominant immunoglobulin produced is IgA. Rarely, lymphoma may arise from this tissue.[2,6]

**Difficulty level: 3**

**16 B** The pathology of ocular cicatricial pemphigoid involves autoantibody production to basement membrane components, resulting in type II hypersensitivity. The subsequent complement activation, inflammatory cell recruitment and cytokine release causes inflammation and eventually scarring and shrinkage of the conjunctiva.[8]

**Difficulty level: 4**

**17 D** Interferons are glycoproteins produced by virus-infected cells, and secreted into the extracellular fluid where they have antiviral effects. Interferon-α is mainly produced by leucocytes, whereas fibroblasts and some other cells produce interferon-β. Interferon-β may be used in the treatment of multiple sclerosis.[6]

**Difficulty level: 3**

**18 C** The MHC is an area on chromosome 6 containing the genes encoding HLA antigens and some complement components. Class I, e.g. HLA-A, B, C, etc., are present on virtually all nucleated cells. When associated with antigen, they indicate to cytotoxic T-cells that the cells should be destroyed. Class II, e.g. HLA-DR, DP, etc., are expressed on B-cells, macrophages and some other cells, and their expression protects against destruction by cytotoxic T-cells.[6]

**Difficulty level: 3**

**19  B**  Graft rejection may be hyperacute (antibody mediated, where circulating antibodies are present to antigens of the graft), acute (cell mediated) or late/chronic. The cornea is an immune privileged site and so rejection will not usually occur unless there is inflammation when this immune privilege is lost. Corneal graft rejection is a type IV hypersensitivity reaction. HLA class matching is not usually required due to the immune privilege, however class I matching has a small beneficial effect on graft survival.[5,7]
**Difficulty level: 3**

**20  B**  The classical pathway is activated by antibody-antigen complexes, such as in SLE. The alternative pathway is activated by the cell walls of Gram-negative bacteria. Both pathways can cleave C3 into C3a and C3b. Opsonisation is mediated by C3b, chemotaxis and inflammation by C3a and C5a, and membrane attack complex by the terminal components C5–C9.[7]
**Difficulty level: 4**

## References

1  Colledge NR, Walker BR, Ralston SH. *Davidson's Principles and Practice of Medicine*. 21st ed. Edinburgh: Churchill Livingstone Elsevier; 2010. (**q1**) p. 133.

2  Kumar V, Abbas A, Fausto N, *et al. Robbins and Cotran Pathologic Basis of Disease*. 8th ed. Philadelphia: Saunders Elsevier; 2010. (**q2**) pp. 343–4, (**q7**) pp. 244–5, (**q15**) p. 778.

3  Rang HP, Dale MM, Ritter JM, *et al. Rang and Dale's Pharmacology*. 7th ed. Edinburgh: Churchill Livingstone Elsevier; 2011. (**q3**) p. 623, (**q6**) pp. 644–5, (**q11**) p. 630, (**q12**) pp. 632–3.

4  Murray PR, Rosenthal KS, Pfaller MA. *Medical Microbiology*. 6th ed. Philadelphia: Mosby Elsevier; 2009. (**q4**) p. 74, (**q10**) pp. 80–1.

5  Kanski JJ. *Clinical Ophthalmology – a systematic approach*. 6th ed. Edinburgh: Butterworth Heinemann Elsevier; 2007. (**q8**) pp. 260–2, (**q9**) pp. 272–3, (**q19**) p. 315.

6  Delves PJ, Martin SJ, Burton DR, *et al. Roitt's Essential Immunology*. 11th ed. Malden: Blackwell; 2006. (**q13**) pp. 19–20, (**q14**) pp. 38–40, 53, (**q15**) p. 163, (**q17**) pp. 17–18, (**q18**) p. 85.

7  Underwood JC, Cross SS. *General and Systematic Pathology*. 5th ed. Edinburgh: Churchill Livingstone Elsevier; 2009. (**q5**) p. 51, (**q19**) pp. 193–5, (**q20**) pp. 173–5.

8  Huang JJ, Gaudio PA. *Ocular Inflammatory Disease and Uveitis Manual: diagnosis & treatment*. Philadelphia: Lippincott Williams & Wilkins; 2010. (**q16**) p. 182.

# 5. Microbiology and immunology ICO answers

**21**  i. T  ii. F  iii. T  iv. T  v. F

Exotoxins may be produced by Gram-positive or -negative bacteria. They include cytolytic enzymes or proteins that impair cell function or cause cell death. Superantigens, such as the toxin produced by *Staphylococcus aureus* in toxic shock syndrome, are a group of toxins that activate large numbers of T-cells, resulting in large amounts of cytokine release and a potentially life-threatening immune reaction. Endotoxins are made by Gram-negative bacteria only and consist of lipopolysaccharide from the bacterial cell wall.[1]
**Difficulty level: 3**


**22**  i. F  ii. T  iii. F  iv. T  v. T

*Pseudomonas* species are Gram-negative rods, and are aerobic bacteria. They possess flagella and pili improving adherence to host cells and also produce exotoxin. Diagnosis can be aided by Gram staining and microscopy and culture on blood or MacConkey agar.

*Pseudomonas* are not able to penetrate healthy corneal epithelium. They are a common cause of corneal ulcers, where the cornea has been breached such as in trauma or hypoxia and are the commonest cause of contact lens-related ulcers.[1]
**Difficulty level: 3**


**23**  i. F  ii. F  iii. F  iv. T  v. T

*Chlamydia* are small Gram-negative microorganisms, which differ from bacteria due to their developmental cycle. They form infectious extracellular elementary bodies which are unable to replicate. In susceptible host cells these are internalised and become reticulate bodies which are able to replicate. *Chlamydia trachomatis* serotypes A–C cause trachoma and serotypes D–K cause oculogenital disease such as adult conjunctivitis and neonatal conjunctivitis. *Chlamydia* infection may present with chronic conjunctivitis.

Polymerase chain reaction (PCR) is the diagnostic investigation of choice.[1,2]
**Difficulty level: 4**

**24**   i. T       ii. F       iii. F       iv. T       v. F

Viruses require the host cell for replication. The binding of viral attachment proteins or other viral surface proteins to host cell surface receptors determines host cell tropism. Once bound to receptors, viral particles are taken up by endocytosis or membrane fusion into the cell and then uncoating of the virus occurs. DNA viruses use host cell RNA polymerase II for transcription to produce messenger RNA. RNA viruses need to encode their own RNA polymerases as the host cell is unable to produce RNA from RNA. Once translation occurs and viral proteins are synthesised, virion assemble occurs and the virus is released from the cell either by cell lysis or budding from the plasma membrane.[1]

**Difficulty level: 3**

**25**   i. T       ii. F       iii. F       iv. T       v. F

Herpes viruses are enveloped double-stranded DNA viruses. Herpes simplex types 1 and 2, herpes zoster, Epstein-Barr virus and *Cytomegalovirus* are examples of herpes viruses. Many herpes viruses can cause latent infection; herpes simplex remains latent within neurones. Most commonly dendritic ulcers are caused by herpes simplex. Both herpes simplex and zoster usually cause anterior segment disease in the eye, but rarely herpes simplex may cause acute retinal necrosis in immunocompetent patients. Herpes zoster may cause progressive outer retinal necrosis in the immunocompromised. Diagnosis is usually made using PCR.[2]

**Difficulty level: 3**

**26**   i. T       ii. F       iii. F       iv. T       v. T

Ganciclovir is a nucleoside analogue and is more effective than aciclovir in the treatment of *Cytomegalovirus* (CMV). It is administered intravenously or intravitreally in the case of CMV retinitis. The major side effect is bone marrow suppression. Foscarnet inhibits viral replication by binding to DNA polymerase to prevent nucleotide binding. It may also be given intravenously or intravitreally, and its major side effect is nephrotoxicity. Aciclovir is only toxic to cells infected by virus and may therefore be used a prophylactic treatment in individuals susceptible to herpetic disease.[2]

**Difficulty level: 4**

**27**    i. F    ii. F    iii. F    iv. T    v. F

Prions are small proteinaceous infectious particles and possess no genome or envelope. They lack antigenicity and produce no immune response or inflammation. Latency periods may be very long before symptoms occur; these are usually due to neurological damage. Prions are resistant to formaldehyde, ionizing radiation and other methods of viral destruction. Autoclaving at 15 psi for 1 hour is effective. Disposable surgical instruments are more commonly used for at-risk procedures for this reason. There is no definitive diagnostic test, but detection of prion protein in a biopsy sample using Western blot is possible.[1]
   **Difficulty level: 4**

**28**    i. F    ii. T    iii. F    iv. F    v. T

HIV is a single-stranded RNA virus. It binds to the CD4 receptor, the co-receptor is either CCR5 or CXCR4. HIV is able to infect any cell with this receptor such as T-cells, macrophages, monocytes and microglial cells of the brain. The single-stranded RNA virus is reverse transcribed to DNA by the viral RNA transcriptase. This is a very error-prone enzyme and thus new strains of virus can be produced. The complementary DNA integrates into the host genome, where it is called the provirus, and is transcribed with cellular genes.[1]
   **Difficulty level: 5**

**29**    i. F    ii. F    iii. F    iv. T    v. F

*Candida* is a yeast-like fungus. It is a commensal organism in 25% to 50% of healthy people. Infection can occur by the patient's own commensal organism if barriers are breached, or by exogenous introduction. *Candida* is a cause of endogenous endophthalmitis in patients with *Candida* sepsis. It can be stained with calcofluor white or cultured on mycologic medium. *Candida* infection of the oesophagus, trachea or lungs is an AIDS-defining illness.[1]
   **Difficulty level: 5**

**30**    i. T    ii. F    iii. F    iv. F    v. T

*Toxoplasma gondii* is an obligate intracellular parasite. The reservoir host is the common house cat and other felines. Transmission is via ingestion of under-cooked meat from animals that may have also been infected (such as pigs) or the orofaecal route via ingestion of contaminated cat faeces. Recurrent inflammation may occur. Chorioretinitis may be associated with a previous scar or be at new site. Severe vitritis may also be a feature. Treatment is only required if the macula, optic nerve or a major blood vessel are threatened. Pyrimethamine and sulphadiazine or clindamycin are common treatments.

It is in *Toxocara canis* that the reservoir host is the dog, and dragging of the optic disc may be seen.[1,2]

**Difficulty level: 3**

**31**  i. F      ii. T      iii. F      iv. F      v. T

Penicillin is a beta-lactam antibiotic and acts by interfering with bacterial cell wall peptidoglycan synthesis. Benzylpenicillin is poorly absorbed by the gastrointestinal tract, whereas amoxicillin is very well absorbed. Amoxicillin is destroyed by beta lactamases produced by *Staphylococcus aureus* and so is not the drug of choice for this infection. Flucloxacillin with or without benzylpenicillin is more commonly used for *S. aureus* infections. Clavulanic acid inhibits beta lactamases and so reduces bacterial resistance to penicillins. Penicillins are excreted by the kidney.[3]

**Difficulty level: 4**

**32**  i. T      ii. T      iii. F      iv. T      v. T

Amphotericin is a macrolide polyene antifungal. It binds to ergosterol in fungal plasma membranes and produces ion channels in them which destroy the membranes' integrity. Amphotericin may be administered intravenously or intravitreally in *Candida* endophthalmitis. The major side effect is nephrotoxicity and so renal function must be monitored. Fluconazole also has good efficacy against *Candida* and has good central nervous system penetration. It may be given intravenously or orally and significant side effects are uncommon.[1]

**Difficulty level: 4**

**33**  i. F      ii. F      iii. T      iv. T      v. T

Syphilis is caused by *Treponema pallidum*, which is a spirochaete. The organism dies quickly on drying or in warm temperature. Ocular features include uveitis, interstitial keratitis, optic neuritis, Argyll Robertson pupils and ocular motor nerve palsies. Treatment is with high-dose penicillin, or doxycyline or erythromycin in penicillin-allergic patients.[2]

**Difficulty level: 3**

**34**   i. T      ii. T      iii. F      iv. F      v. T

IgG is the commonest immunoglobulin, and is often found in extravascular fluids, where it acts to neutralise toxins and fix complement via the C1 pathway. IgG also facilitates binding to phagocytic cells. IgA plays a role in the defence of mucous membranes and is present in their secretions. IgM is a large, mainly intravascular molecule. It plays a role early in the immune response and activates complement-dependent cell lysis. IgD is present on the surface of lymphocytes and probably acts as an antigen receptor. IgE is bound to mast cells and is important in the response to parasitic infections as well as playing a role in atopy.[4]
  **Difficulty level: 3**


**35**   i. T      ii. T      iii. T      iv. F      v. T

Complement activation leads to the attraction of phagocytic cells to and cytolysis of microbes. Complement fixes antibody bound to antigen via the classical pathway. Both the classical and alternative pathways are able to cleave C3. Opsonisation is mediated by C3b, chemotaxis and inflammation by C3a and C5a, and membrane attack complex causing cytolysis by the terminal components C5–C9.
  T-cell activation occurs when the T-cell receptor binds to antigen presented in association with MHC.[4]
  **Difficulty level: 3**


**36**   i. F      ii. T      iii. T      iv. T      v. F

T-cells are unable to process free antigen and respond to those presented via MHC. MHC class I is present on almost all cells, and present antigen that is endogenously produced such as viral products from an infected cell. Cytotoxic T-cells respond to antigen presented via MHC class I, resulting in cell destruction. Dendritic cells, macrophages and B cells are examples of antigen presenting cells (APC). They process and present exogenously synthesised antigen (eg. bacterial products) via MHC class II. Helper T-cells are activated as a result of antigen presentation via APCs.[5]
  **Difficulty level: 3**

**37**   i. T       ii. T       iii. T       iv. F       v. F

The ocular surface is protected by components of the innate and adaptive immune system. Components of the innate immune system include lysozyme (effective against Gram-negative bacteria), lactoferrin and complement (effective against Gram-positive bacteria), tear lipid which has an antibacterial effect and polymorphonuclear leucocytes. Components of the adaptive immune system include IgA, MALT and dendritic cells.[6]
   **Difficulty level: 3**

**38**   i. F       ii. T       iii. T       iv. T       v. F

TNF-α is produced by T-helper cells and is a feature of all types of uveitis including granulomatous and HLA-B27 related anterior uveitis. TNF-α also activates neutrophils, causes fever and induces tissue destruction. Infliximab and adalimumab are both TNF-α inhibitors. Infliximab may cause reactivation of infections and so it is essential to perform a chest X-ray to exclude tuberculosis before commencing therapy. Infliximab is a strong immunosuppressant and is effective in treating all types of uveitis, but is usually reserved for cases that have not responded to steroid therapy.[7]
   **Difficulty level: 4**

**39**   i. F       ii. T       iii. F       iv. T       v. F

Positive c-ANCA antibodies are associated with Wegener's granulomatosis. Anti-Ro and La antibodies are associated with Sjögren's syndrome and less commonly with systemic lupus erythematosus. Anti-TSH receptor antibodies are associated with Graves' disease. Anti-acetylcholine receptor antibodies are associated with myasthenia gravis. Anti-double-stranded DNA antibodies are associated with systemic lupus erythematosus.[4]
   **Difficulty level: 3**

**40**   i. T       ii. F       iii. F       iv. T       v. T

Cytokines are low molecular weight proteins and regulate the duration and size of the inflammatory response. They are therefore produced in a transient manner and act locally in a paracrine fashion. Cytokines often have multiple effects and act via cell surface receptors to change patterns of RNA and protein expression. IL-1 is produced by macrophages and fibroblasts and has many actions including the proliferation of activated B- and T-cells, induction of

fever and other acute phase proteins, as well as the induction of prostaglandins and other cytokines. TNF-α is produced by T-helper cells and macrophages.[4]
**Difficulty level: 3**

## References

1 Murray PR, Rosenthal KS, Pfaller MA. *Medical Microbiology*. 6th ed. Philadelphia: Mosby Elsevier; 2009. (**q21**) pp. 182–3, (**q22**) pp. 336–7, (**q23**) pp. 442–3, (**q24**) pp. 45–55, (**q27**) pp. 661–5, (**q28**) pp. 630–2, (**q29**) pp. 757–9, (**q30**) pp. 841–4, (**q32**) pp. 701–5.

2 Kanski JJ. *Clinical Ophthalmology – a systematic approach*. 6th ed. Edinburgh: Butterworth Heinemann Elsevier; 2007. (**q23**) pp. 221–2, (**q25**) pp. 262, 280, (**q26**) p. 477, (**q30**) pp. 469–72, (**q33**) pp. 891–2.

3 Rang HP, Dale MM, Ritter JM, *et al. Rang and Dale's Pharmacology*. 7th ed. Edinburgh: Churchill Livingstone Elsevier; 2011. (**q31**) pp. 625–7.

4 Delves P, Martin S, Burton D, *et al. Essential Immunology*. 11th ed. Malden: Wiley Blackwell; 2006. (**q34**) pp. 59–60, (**q35**) p. 20, (**q39**) p. 414, (**q40**) pp. 187, 209.

5 Kumar V, Abbas A, Fausto N, *et al. Robbins and Cotran Pathologic Basis of Disease*. 8th ed. Philadelphia: Saunders Elsevier; 2010. (**q36**) pp. 190–5.

6 Forrester J, Dick A, McMenamin A, *et al. The Eye: basic sciences in practice*. 2nd ed. Philadelphia: Saunders Elsevier; 2007. (**q37**) p. 355.

7 Heiligenhaus A, Thurau S, Hennig M. Anti-inflammatory treatment of uveitis with biologicals: new treatment options that reflect pathogenetic knowledge of the disease. *Graefes Arch Clin Exp Ophthalmol*. 2010; **248**: 1531–51 (**q38**).

# 6. Embryology and development FRCOphth answers

1 **C** The corneal and conjunctival epithelium, caruncle, lids including cilia and glands of Moll, Zeis and Meibom, lens, lacrimal gland and drainage system are derived from surface ectoderm. Striated muscle fibres and endothelium of blood vessels are derived from mesoderm.[1]
**Difficulty level: 3**

2 **B** Bergmeister's papilla consists of old vessels and glial strands project-ing forwards from the optic disc representing the former hyaloid artery.

Remnants of the anterior attachment of the hyaloid artery on the posterior lens capsule is called Mittendorf's dot.[2]
**Difficulty level: 4**

3   **A**   During the third month of development the outer neuroblastic layer forms bipolar cells, horizontal cells and the nuclei of rods and cones. The inner neuroblastic layer forms ganglion cells, amacrine cells and nuclei of Müller cells.[1]
**Difficulty level: 4**

4   **A**   The ciliary body epithelium is derived from neuroectoderm.[1]
**Difficulty level: 3**

5   **C**   Failure of closure of the optic fissure during the fifth week of gestation leads to defects of the iris, ciliary body, choroid, optic nerve and closely associated structures. Typically these anomalies occur inferiorly, although in atypical colobomas they can occur in other positions. Lid colobomas are not related to failure of optic fissure closure.[1]
**Difficulty level: 3**

6   **C**   Remnants of the hyaloid system are part of the primary vitreous. The secondary vitreous eventually becomes the main vitreous body. The tertiary vitreous is most peripherally located and involved with the development of zonules. Quaternary vitreous does not exist![2]
**Difficulty level: 4**

7   **D**   The ophthalmic artery, temporal long posterior ciliary artery, short posterior ciliary arteries and central retinal artery can be traced to the dorsal ophthalmic artery. The ventral ophthalmic artery develops into the nasal long posterior ciliary artery.[2]
**Difficulty level: 4**

8   **A**   The maxillary branch of the trigeminal nerve derives from the upper part of the first pharyngeal arch. The mandibular branch of the trigeminal nerve is derived from the lower part of the first pharyngeal arch.[2]
**Difficulty level: 4**

9   **C**   The iris sphincter and dilator muscles and bilayered iris epithelium are derived from neuroectoderm.[1]
**Difficulty level: 3**

**10 B** The optic vesicle is formed by a lateral out-pouching from the diencephalon.[2]
**Difficulty level: 4**

**11 C** The neural tube forms on day 22 post-conception. The optic pits first appear on day 23. The optic vesicle is fully formed by day 25. The optic cup appears on day 27. The optic/embryonic fissure closes on day 33 (fifth week).[2]
**Difficulty level: 4**

**12 B** Approximate correlation of embryonic length with gestational age:[2]
Day 22  : 2 mm
Day 27  : 5 mm
Day 29  : 7 mm
Day 37  : 9 mm
Day 44  : 15 mm
**Difficulty level: 3**

**13 A** The final diameter of the cornea is determined by the diameter of the optic cup.[1]
**Difficulty level: 3**

**14 C** At term, a single layer of ganglion cells is present as an internal nuclear layer overlying macula cones. These are displaced by the fourth to sixth month of life. Because cones are not fully developed until several months after birth, the newborn infant has imperfect central fixation.[1]
**Difficulty level: 4**

**15 B** In terms of developmental milestones, a 3-month-old baby should have control of head movements, be able to grasp objects and fix and follow. A 6-month-old can roll over, sit up, play with their toes and babble. At 12 months of age, one would expect the infant to crawl, pick up objects and oppose fingers to thumb. At 18 months, one would expect the child to be able to walk, stack blocks and scribble with a crayon.[3]
**Difficulty level: 2**

**16 B** Observing ability to fix and follow is useful in infants less than 3 months of age. Forced-choice preferential looking methods (e.g. Cardiff cards) are useful in preverbal children. From about 2 years of age Kay's pictures may be appropriate. Snellen or LogMAR charts can be used in cooperative children from age 5 years onwards.[4]
**Difficulty level: 2**

**17  A**  Optokinetic nystagmus offers only a gross assessment of ability to perceive visual stimuli. Forced-choice preferential looking tests have a tendency to overestimate visual acuity in amblyopes. Single optotype tests again tend to overestimate visual acuity in amblyopes as the phenomenon of crowding is removed.[4]
**Difficulty level: 3**

**18  C**  With maternal rubella in the first trimester, the most common ocular abnormality in the foetus is cataract, which is bilateral in 75% of cases. Other anomalies associated are nystagmus, microphthalmos, retinopathy and infantile glaucoma. Acute conjunctivitis is common early in the course of measles. The most common ocular complication of mumps is dacroadenitis.[5]
**Difficulty level: 3**

**19  B**  The ultimate size of the eyeball is reached at 8 years of age. It is shorter in anteroposterior diameter at birth, making the eye relatively hypermetropic.[2]
**Difficulty level: 3**

**20  B**  The *Bcl-2* gene codes for a family of proteins which inhibit apoptosis. The *p53* gene codes for a tumour-suppression protein which activates DNA fragmentation and apoptosis. The *BAX* and *Fas* genes induce apoptosis.[2]
**Difficulty level: 4**

## References

1  Snell R, Lemp M. *Clinical Anatomy of the Eye*. 2nd ed. Malden: Blackwell Publishing; 2006. (**q1**) pp. 14–15, (**q3**) p. 4, (**q4**) p. 9, (**q5**) p. 18, (**q9**) p. 12, (**q13**) p. 13, (**q14**) p. 7.

2  Chalam KV, editor. *Fundamentals and Principles of Ophthalmology. Part II: Embryology*. San Francisco: American Academy of Ophthalmology Basic and Clinical Science Course 2010–2011. (**q2**) p. 51, (**q6**) p. 58, (**q7**) p. 64, (**q8**) p. 71, (**q10**) p. 50, (**q11**) p. 51, (**q12**) p. 52, (**q19**) p. 74, (**q20**) p. 156.

3  Lissauer T, Clayden G. *Illustrated Textbook of Paediatrics*. 2nd ed. Philadelphia: Mosby Elsevier; 2003. (**q15**) pp. 24–8.

4  Sundaram V, Barsam A, Alwitry A, *et al*. *Training in Ophthalmology: the essential clinical curriculum*. Oxford: Oxford University Press; 2008. (**q16, q17**) p. 328.

5  Kanski JJ. *Clinical Ophthalmology – a systematic approach*. 6th ed. Edinburgh: Butterworth Heinemann Elsevier; 2007. (**q18**) p. 900.

# 6. Embryology and development ICO answers

**21**   i. T      ii. T      iii. F      iv. F      v. T

Fibres of the extraocular muscles derive from mesoderm. Sphincter and dilator pupillae muscles derive from neuroectoderm. Ciliary muscles derive from neural crest cells.[1]

**Difficulty level: 3**

**22**   i. T      ii. F      iii. F      iv. F      v. T

The muscular and connective tissue layers of all ocular and orbital vessels derive from neural crest cells. The endothelial lining of all ocular and orbital vessels derive from neural crest cells. The primitive dorsal ophthalmic artery becomes the definitive ophthalmic artery. The primitive ventral ophthalmic artery almost disappears; only a portion remains as the long posterior nasal ciliary artery. Vascularisation of the nasal retina is complete before that of the temporal retina because of the shorter distance from the optic disc to the nasal ora serrata. This has implications for the presentation in retinopathy of prematurity.[1]

**Difficulty level: 4**

**23**   i. T      ii. F      iii. F      iv. T      v. F

The primary vitreous forms in the first month of development. Iris pigmentation takes place in the second trimester. Development of choroidal melanocytes occurs at this time. The eyelids fuse at the end of the second month and open in the third trimester. The ciliary body can be identified from the third month of development. Formation of the extraocular muscles occurs in third trimester.[1]

**Difficulty level: 4**

**24**   i.  F       ii.  T       iii.  T       iv.  T       v.  T

At birth, the baby can fix and follow objects in the midline. Preference for patterned objects over plain ones can also be demonstrated at birth. The ability to move their head to continue fixing develops by 6 weeks.[2]
   **Difficulty level: 2**

**25**   i.  T       ii.  T       iii.  F       iv.  F       v.  T

The cornea is composed of surface ectoderm which forms the corneal epithelium and neural crest cells which form Bowman's layer, stroma, Descemet's membrane and endothelium. The diameter of the cornea measures 2 mm at 12 weeks gestation, 4.5 mm at 17 weeks and over 9 mm at 35 weeks. Bowman's layer is the last of the five corneal layers to form.[1]
   **Difficulty level: 4**

**26**   i.  F       ii.  F       iii.  T       iv.  T       v.  F

The outer layer of the optic cup develops into the RPE. The inner layer develops into the neurosensory retina. The inner neuroblastic layer gives rise to ganglion cells, Müller cells and amacrine cells. The outer neuroblastic gives rise to the bipolar cells and rods and cones. It is estimated that the eye first becomes sensitive to light at the seventh month of foetal life. Colour sense develops in the second year.[1]
   **Difficulty level: 3**

**27**   i.  T       ii.  T       iii.  F       iv.  F       v.  F

The lacrimal gland and lacrimal drainage system develop from buried buds of surface ectoderm. The lacrimal gland begins to develop at the eighth week. However, the gland does not begin to secrete tears until about 1 month after birth, explaining why newly born babies do not produce tears when born. The lacrimal drainage system opens in the second and third trimesters. The distal portion of the nasolacrimal duct is the last to open and is a common site for tear duct obstruction in the infant.[1]
   **Difficulty level: 3**

**28**   i. T      ii. T      iii. T      iv. F      v. F

Corneal epithelium derives from surface ectoderm. Retinal pigment epithelium derives from neuroectoderm.[1]
   **Difficulty level: 2**

**29**   i. T      ii. T      iii. T      iv. F      v. F

In amblyopia there is no demonstrable abnormality of the optic pathways. Anisometropic amblyopia may coexist with strabismic amblyopia. Stimulus deprivation amblyopia occurs when no image or a degraded image forms at the fovea.[3]
   **Difficulty level: 1**

**30**   i. T      ii. T      iii. T      iv. F      v. T

Since the secondary vitreous is secreted by the retina this accounts for the relatively firm attachment of the vitreous to the internal limiting membrane in early life. Tertiary vitreous is secreted from neural ectoderm of the ciliary body, forming zonular fibres which attach to the equator of the lens capsule.[1]
   **Difficulty level: 2**

**31**   i. F      ii. T      iii. T      iv. T      v. F

The macula area develops initially as an increase in the ganglion cell layer temporal to the disc just after midterm. During the seventh month there is peripheral displacement of the ganglion cells leaving a central depression, the fovea centralis. Adaptation of cone inner and outer segments allows increased foveal density. At birth, the ganglion cells have been reduced to a single layer at the fovea. By 4 months of age the cone nuclei in the centre of the fovea have no ganglion cells covering them. The reason for the newborn's imperfect central fixation is that the cones do not fully develop until several months after birth.[4]
   **Difficulty level: 3**

**32**　i. T　　ii. T　　iii. F　　iv. F　　v. T

The central retinal artery enters the optic stalk approximately 10 mm posterior to the retina. In the second and third months of embryogenesis, nerve fibres from the ganglion cells pass into the optic stalk forming the optic nerve.[1]
　　**Difficulty level: 3**

**33**　i. T　　ii. F　　iii. T　　iv. F　　v. T

The brain and eye develop from the most anterior region of the neural plate. The neural folds begin to close to form the neural tube at the 3rd week of gestation.[5]
　　**Difficulty level: 4**

**34**　i. T　　ii. T　　iii. T　　iv. F　　v. T

The trabecular meshwork derives from neural crest cells.[1]
　　**Difficulty level: 3**

**35**　i. T　　ii. T　　iii. T　　iv. T　　v. F

The central retinal artery supplies the inner layers of the retina down to and including the inner nuclear layer of the retina.[5]
　　**Difficulty level: 2**

**36**　i. T　　ii. F　　iii. T　　iv. F　　v. F

The lens placode is first seen at day 22 of gestation. The first suture marking the foetal nucleus is shaped like a Y anteriorly and inverted Y posteriorly. The hyaloid artery and tunica vascular lentis regress before birth. For its nutrition, the lens is dependent upon diffusion from the aqueous and vitreous humours.[1]
　　**Difficulty level: 2**

**37**　i. T　　ii. T　　iii. T　　iv. T　　v. T

The developmental gene *PAX6* is located at 11p13. The *PAX6* gene product is a transcription factor needed for development of the eye. For example, it induces differentiation of progenitor cells into neurones in the retina as well as expression of crystallins in lens epithelial cells. A mutation in a different homeobox gene may cause a similar clinical manifestation, e.g. *RIEG1* also results in Peters' anomaly.[1]

**Difficulty level: 3**

---

**38**   i. T      ii. T      iii. T      iv. F      v. F

The pigmented iris epithelium and iris muscles derive from neuroectoderm. The connective tissue of iris and ciliary ganglion derive from neural crest cells.[1]

**Difficulty level: 3**

---

**39**   i. T      ii. F      iii. F      iv. T      v. F

Myelination starts at the chiasm and progresses towards the lamina cribosa. Myelination of the optic nerve starts in the seventh month of gestation and is completed about 1 month after birth. The retinal nerve fibre layer is not myelinated. However, if there is failure of the myelination process to stop at the lamina cribosa, myelinated nerve fibre layers can be seen in the retina.[4]

**Difficulty level: 2**

---

**40**   i. F      ii. T      iii. F      iv. F      v. T

Early in development the eyeball develops at a faster rate than the orbit, so by the sixth month of foetal life the anterior half of the eyeball projects beyond the orbital opening. The medial wall forms from the lateral nasal process. The lateral and inferior walls develop from the maxillary process. The optic axes are initially directed laterally towards the side of the head (180 degrees) in the second month and then move more anteriorly, reaching 105 degrees in the third month, 71 degrees at birth and 68 degrees in adulthood.[4]

**Difficulty level: 4**

## References

1 Chalam KV, editor. *Fundamentals and Principles of Ophthalmology. Part II: Embryology*. San Francisco: American Academy of Ophthalmology Basic and Clinical Science Course 2010–2011. **(q21)** p. 53, **(q22)** p. 61, **(q23)** p. 72, **(q25)** p. 57, **(q26)** p. 64, **(q27)** p. 78, **(q28)** p. 73, **(q30)** p. 51, **(q32)** p. 58, **(q34)** p. 62, **(q36)** p. 63, **(q37)** p. 64, **(q38)** p. 69.

2 Lissauer T, Clayden G. *Illustrated Textbook of Paediatrics*. 2nd ed. Philadelphia: Mosby Elsevier; 2003. **(q24)** pp. 24–8.

3 Sundaram V, Barsam A, Alwitry A, *et al*. *Training in Ophthalmology: the essential clinical curriculum*. Oxford: Oxford University Press; 2008. (**q29**) p. 334.

4 Snell R, Lemp M. *Clinical Anatomy of the Eye*. 2nd ed. Malden: Blackwell Publishing; 2006. (**q31, q39**) p. 7, (**q40**) p. 15.

5 Forrester J, Dick A, McMenamin A, *et al*. *The Eye: basic sciences in practice*. 2nd ed. Philadelphia: Saunders Elsevier; 2007. (**q33**) pp. 99–101, (**q35**) p. 112.

# 7. Optics FRCOphth answers

1 **C** One complete oscillation refers to a cycle. The maximum displacement of an imaginary particle on the wave from the baseline is amplitude. Any portion of a cycle is called a phase.[1]
**Difficulty level: 2**

2 **C** If two waves with the same amplitude are half a cycle out of phase, they cancel each other out, which is termed destructive interference. In low-reflection lens coatings, light reflected from the superficial layer and that from the deep surface cancel each other out, reducing reflectance. In the corneal stroma, collagen bundles are spaced in order to minimise transmission of any deviated light as this is eliminated by destructive interference. Photochromic lenses change their transmission characteristics based on the intensity of incident light and do not use the principle of interference.[1]
**Difficulty level: 3**

3 **C** Pelli-Robson is a test of contrast sensitivity and displays letters on backgrounds with reducing levels of contrast. The Titmus test assesses 3000 to 40 seconds of arc, the Frisby test 600 to 15 seconds of arc, and the TNO test 480 to 25 seconds of arc.[1]
**Difficulty level: 3**

4 **A** The intensity of light emitted from a source is radiant intensity, the amount of light falling on a surface is irradiance and the amount of light reflected from a surface is radiance.[1]
**Difficulty level: 4**

5 **B** Lumen is the unit for luminous flux, candelas (lumen per steradian) for luminous intensity and Watts per steradian for radiant intensity.[1]
**Difficulty level: 4**

**6**  **C**  The image of an object formed by reflection at a plane surface is erect, virtual, laterally inverted and lies as far behind the surface as the object is in front of it.[1]
**Difficulty level: 2**

**7**  **D**  Images formed from the reflecting surfaces of the eye are termed catoptric images. These surfaces are the anterior (I) and posterior (II) corneal surfaces and the anterior (III) and posterior (IV) lens surfaces. Images I, II and III are erect and virtual. Image IV is real and inverted.[1]
**Difficulty level: 3**

**8**  **D**  When light passes into a denser medium, the wavelength decreases as does the velocity.[1]
**Difficulty level: 3**

**9**  **C**  Total internal reflection is used in prisms, fibre-optic cables and also occurs at the angle of the anterior chamber and peripheral retina of the eye.[1]
**Difficulty level: 3**

**10**  **D**  An object located between the centre of curvature and principal focus of a concave mirror has an image that is real, enlarged, inverted and lies outside the centre of curvature.[1]
**Difficulty level: 3**

**11**  **B**  The angle of deviation of a ray of light when refracted by a prism is determined by the refractive index of the material of which the prism is made, the refracting angle of the prism and the angle of incidence of the ray. The angle of deviation is least when the angle of incidence equals the angle of emergence.[1]
**Difficulty level: 3**

**12**  **A**  The image formed by a prism is erect, virtual and displaced towards the apex of the prism.[1]
**Difficulty level: 3**

**13**  **B**  For a glass prism of refractive index 1.5:

Angle of deviation (D) = refracting angle ($\alpha$)/2

Therefore, 1 prism dioptre power produces an angle of deviation of 0.5 degrees, and a 20-dioptre powered prism deviates light through 10 degrees.[1]
**Difficulty level: 3**

**14 D** For a convex lens, placing an object inside the first principal focus ($F_1$) results in an image that is enlarged, erect and virtual and further from the lens than the object.[1]
**Difficulty level: 3**

**15 C** Prismatic power = lens power × decentration (in cm)
Decentration of a concave lens temporally results in a base-in prism, and nasally results in base out.[1]
**Difficulty level: 3**

**16 B** To calculate the spherical equivalent, add the spherical power and half the cylindrical power.[1]
**Difficulty level: 3**

**17 C** Add the power of the sphere and cylinder to give the power of the new sphere, e.g. (–4) + (–3) = –7. Change the sign of the cylinder and rotate by 90 degrees to give the new cylinder.[1]
**Difficulty level: 3**

**18 A** Toric formula =

$$\frac{\text{Surface power of sphere}}{\text{Surface power and axis of base curve/surface power and axis of cylinder}}$$

- Transpose prescription so cylinder and base curve are of same sign
- To obtain spherical power, algebraically subtract base curve from original sphere e.g. +2 – (–2) = 4
- Axis of base curve is 90 degrees to cylinder
- Cylindrical power is sum of base curve, i.e. (–2) + (–1) = –3 and original cylindrical power, i.e. 180 degrees[1]

**Difficulty level: 5**

**19 C** Spherical aberrations occur since the rays passing through the periphery of a lens are deviated more than those passing through the central part. Within the eye, to minimise spherical aberration, the anterior corneal surface is flatter peripherally than centrally (i.e. aplanatic); the nucleus of the lens has a higher refractive index than the periphery and so has more of an effect; and the iris acts as a stop so that only the paraxial area of the lens is used. Pantoscopic tilt is used to minimise oblique astigmatism.[1]
**Difficulty level: 3**

**20 D** Barrel distortion occurs with high minus (i.e. concave) lenses. Image magnification, pin-cushion distortion and ring scotoma due to prismatic effect of the lens edge are all problems with spectacle correction of

aphakia. The jack-in-the-box effect may also occur with ring scotoma as position of the scotoma changes with eye movement, so objects may disappear into or appear out of the scotoma.[1]
**Difficulty level: 3**

21  **A**  The principal point (P) is at 1.35 mm behind the anterior corneal surface, the nodal point (N) at 7.08 mm, first focal point at –15.7 mm and second focal point at 24.13 mm.[1]
**Difficulty level: 3**

22  **A**  The crystalline lens has an effective power of 15 dioptres when in situ. The cornea has a refractive power of 43 dioptres.[1]
**Difficulty level: 2**

23  **D**  The dioptric power of the eye at rest is the static refraction, and that when fully accommodated is its dynamic refraction.[1]
**Difficulty level: 2**

24  **B**  The AC/A ratio is the number of prism dioptres of convergence which accompanies 1 dioptre of accommodation – the normal range is 3 : 1 to 5 : 1. A high AC/A ratio may be associated with convergence excess esotropia, where the eyes are straight for distance but an esotropia is seen for near focus due to excess convergence. Conditions A and D do not exist.[1]
**Difficulty level: 2**

25  **B**  Ametropia may be due to problems with axial length (i.e. the eye being too long or short to bring the image into focus on the retina) or refractive problems (i.e. increased or reduced refractive power of the eye). In keratoconus the corneal refractive power is higher than normal, causing refractive myopia. This may also be caused by nucleosclerotic cataract, in which the refractive power of the lens increases.[1]
**Difficulty level: 3**

26  **D**  In simple astigmatism, one ray of light comes into focus on the retina, and the light from the other meridian in front (myopic astigmatism) or behind (hypermetropic astigmatism) it. In compound hypermetropic astigmatism, light from all meridians comes into focus behind the retina.[1]
**Difficulty level: 3**

27  **B**  In a hypermetropic eye, by moving a convex lens away from the eye the effectivity of the lens is decreased. The converse is true in myopic patients: moving a correcting concave lens away from the eye reduces its

effectivity, so a stronger lens is required. Therefore documentation of the back vertex distance (that from the front of the eye to the posterior lens surface) is important when prescribing glasses for high myopes.[1]
**Difficulty level: 3**

**28 C** The new lens power can be calculated by the formula:

$$F_2 = \frac{F_1}{1 - dF_1}$$

Where $F_1$ is the power of the lens required in the old position, and d is the distance moved in metres (d has a positive sign if the lens is moved towards the eye, and negative sign if the lens is moved away from the eye).[1]
**Difficulty level: 4**

**29 A** SRK formula:
Lens power = A constant – (axial length × 2.5) – (average K readings × 0.9)[1]
**Difficulty level: 4**

**30 C** Progressive addition or varifocal lenses have lens powers that gradually change from distance to near correction across the lens. Between the distance and near visual points is the progression corridor. Narrow progression corridors are difficult to tolerate. Newer designs aim to have wide progression corridors. Lenses with smaller distance and near portions ('soft' designs) allow for a wider progression corridor.[1]
**Difficulty level: 3**

## Reference

1 Elkington AR, Frank HJ, Greaney MJ. *Clinical Optics*. 3rd ed. Oxford: Blackwell Publishing; 2006. (**q1**) p. 8, (**q2**) p. 9, (**q3**) pp. 16, 19–20, (**q4**) pp. 20–1, (**q5**) pp. 21–3, (**q6**) p. 27, (**q7**) pp. 111–12, (**q8**) p. 34, (**q9**) pp. 38–9, (**q10**) p. 30, (**q11**) pp. 43–4, (**q12, q13**) p. 44, (**q14**) p. 58, (**q15**) pp. 64–5, (**q16**) p. 71, (**q17**) p. 76, (**q18**) p. 78, (**q19**) pp. 92–3, (**q20**) pp. 130–1, (**q21, q22**) p. 105, (**q23**) p. 109, (**q24**) pp. 110–11, (**q25**) p. 113, (**q26**) p. 115, (**q27, 28**) pp. 121–3, (**q29**) p. 136, (**q30**) pp. 150–1.

# 7. Optics ICO answers

**31**  i. T  ii. T  iii. T  iv. F  v. T

Up to 3 prism dioptres may be incorporated into corneal contact lenses, but because the weight of the prism rotates the lens, the prism is always base down, and thus can only correct vertical strabismus. Special scleral contact lenses may correct vertical or horizontal strabismus of up to 6 dioptres divided between the two lenses.[1]
   **Difficulty level: 3**

**32**  i. T  ii. F  iii. F  iv. F  v. T

In a Galilean telescope a convex objective lens and concave eyepiece lens are used and the lenses are separated by the sum of their focal lengths. For example, a convex lens of 2.5 dioptres has focal length of 40 cm, so when used with a concave lens of –10 dioptres which has a focal length of –10 cm, would be separated by 30 cm (i.e. the sum of their focal lengths: 40 + (–10) = 30 cm). It produces an erect, enlarged image. An astronomical telescope uses two convex lenses.[1]
   **Difficulty level: 4**

**33**  i. T  ii. T  iii. F  iv. T  v. F

Reduced field of view, reduced depth of focus, the need to be held close to the patient's eye and unsteadiness of the patient's hand are all factors that may limit usefulness of magnifiers as low visual aids. The need to be held close and unsteadiness of the hand may be overcome by spectacle mounting of low visual aids. Field of view may be increased by using an inverted Galilean telescope (concave objective lens and convex eye piece lens).[1]
   **Difficulty level: 3**

**34**  i. F  ii. F  iii. F  iv. T  v. T

Thermokeratoplasty is used in the treatment of hypermetropia: focal burns are used to cause contraction of corneal collagen, thus increasing curvature and corneal power. Photorefractive keratotomy and radial keratotomy, where an excimer laser or partial thickness incisions respectively, are used to change the anterior corneal curvature and are used to treat lesser degrees of myopia, but the best results are obtained in cases of 5–6 dioptres or lower amounts of myopia.[1]

**Difficulty level: 3**

**35**   i. F      ii. T      iii. T      iv. F      v. T

In an aphakic eye, the convex anterior surface of the silicone oil acts as a powerful convex lens. This increases the refractive power of the eye resulting in myopia. In a phakic patient, the higher refractive index of silicone oil compared to the lens changes the posterior surface of the lens from a converging to a diverging surface. This causes hypermetropia.

A gas bubble in a phakic eye increases the power of the posterior surface of the lens, causing myopic shift. In an aphakic eye, gas causes a hypermetropic shift. Use of scleral buckles can compress the globe which causes astigmatism and increases axial length causing myopia.[1]

**Difficulty level: 4**

**36**   i. F      ii. T      iii. T      iv. F      v. F

Light of wavelength 400–1400 nm is transmitted through the ocular media to the retina: this includes visible light (400–780 nm) and near-infrared rays. UVB and UVC light is absorbed by the cornea and sclera, and UVA light by the lens. The genes for red and green opsins are on the X chromosome, the blue cone opsin gene is on chromosome 7. Deuteranopia, protanopia and tritanopia are an absence of green, red and blue cone function respectively. Deuteranomaly, protanomaly and tritanomaly indicate a shift in green, red and blue cone sensitivity respectively.[1]

**Difficulty level: 3**

**37**   i. F      ii. T      iii. F      iv. T      v. F

Fluorescence is the property of a molecule to spontaneously emit light of a longer wavelength when stimulated by light of a shorter wavelength. Fluorescein emits yellow-green light of wavelength 520–530 nm when stimulated by blue light (465–490 nm). A polarised beam of light is one in which the individual wave motions lie parallel to each other. Birefringent substances transmit light waves lying parallel to their structure but redirect light waves that are perpendicular. For example, amyloid plaques exhibit apple-green birefringence when viewed under polarised light. Dichroic substances absorb light waves not aligned with their structure, and so all that exits is a beam of polarised light.[1]

**Difficulty level: 3**

**38    i. T        ii. T        iii. T        iv. F        v. F**

The image formed when light is reflected in a convex mirror is virtual, erect, diminished and laterally inverted. These features are true irrespective of the distance between the object and the mirror. For concave mirrors the image is inverted if located outside the centre of curvature or between the centre of curvature and principal focus; it is erect if located within the principal focus of a concave mirror.[1]

**Difficulty level: 3**

**39    i. T        ii. T        iii. F        iv. F        v. T**

Regarding the refraction of light at a curved surface, Snell's law is obeyed. This states that the incident ray, refracted ray and normal all lie in the same plane; and that the angles of incidence and refraction are related to the refractive index of the medium.

If the refractive index of the medium the light enters into is higher than the original medium, light is converged to a focus. If the refractive index of the medium the light enters into is lower than the original medium, light is diverged. The surface refracting power of a curved surface is inversely proportional to its radius of curvature, and these are related by the formula:

Surface power = $(n_2 - n_1)/r$

where $n_1$ and $n_2$ are the refractive indices of the first and second medium respectively and r is the radius of curvature of the surface in metres.

Surface power is given a negative sign for diverging surfaces and a positive sign for converging surfaces.[1]

**Difficulty level: 3**

**40    i. F        ii. T        iii. T        iv. F        v. F**

In the Prentice position, one surface of the prism is perpendicular to the incident ray of light. In the position of minimum deviation, the angle of incidence is equal to the angle of emergence. In the Prentice position, deviation is greater than in the position of minimum deviation. The Prentice position power is normally specified for glass prisms such as in trial lenses; the position of minimum deviation is that specified for plastic prisms such as in prism bars.

The refractive index of glass is 1.5. The refractive power of prisms stacked on top of one another is *not* the same as the sum of the refractive powers of the individual prisms as the light entering the second prism will not be at the correct angle. However, a horizontal and vertical prism may be stacked. A prism of power 2 prism dioptres deviates light through 1 degree.[1]
**Difficulty level: 3**

**41**  i.  F      ii.  F      iii.  T      iv.  T      v.  T

Fresnel prisms are temporary plastic prisms stuck onto the surface of spectacle lenses. They can be used in squint due to cranial nerve palsy where the deviation is likely to change. When prescribing prisms, the correction is usually divided between both spectacle lenses. The apex of the prisms is placed in the direction of deviation of the eye. Base-out prisms are used to treat convergence insufficiency to build up the patient's fusional reserve – they are not worn all the time. Prisms may be used to assess cases of fictitious blindness, as a seeing eye will move to regain fixation if a prism is placed in front of it.[1]
**Difficulty level: 3**

**42**  i.  T      ii.  T      iii.  T      iv.  T      v.  F

The image formed by a thin concave lens is virtual, erect and smaller than the object and positioned between the second principal focus and the lens. It is not laterally inverted.[1]
**Difficulty level: 3**

**43**  i.  T      ii.  F      iii.  F      iv.  T      v.  T

The peripheral part of a spherical lens acts as a prism when light is incident on it. Prism power can be calculated by the following formula:

Prism power = F × D

where F is lens power in dioptres and D is decentration in centimetres. When a concave lens is decentred nasally, a base-out prism results.[1]
**Difficulty level: 3**

**44**  i.  F      ii.  F      iii.  T      iv.  F      v.  F

The Maddox rod is used to test extraocular muscle balance and is composed of several powerful convex cylindrical lenses. When a white point source of light placed more than 6 metres away is viewed through a Maddox rod, the image seen is a line that is perpendicular to the cylinders in the Maddox rod. Incident light that is parallel to the cylinders in the Maddox rod are undeviated and brought to focus on the retina. Incident light that is perpendicular to the cylinders in the Maddox rod is brought to focus between the Maddox rod and the retina and therefore not seen as an image.[1]

**Difficulty level: 3**

**45**   i. T      ii. F      iii. F      iv. F      v. T

A lens whose cylindrical surface is curved in both the horizontal and vertical meridians is called a toric lens. The principal meridian of minimum curvature is called the base curve. Each meridian of curvature forms a separate line focus; the distance between these is called the interval of Sturm. The spherical equivalent is calculated by adding the spherical power and half of the cylindrical power.[1]

**Difficulty level: 3**

**46**   i. F      ii. T      iii. T      iv. F      v. F

When a convex lens is placed over a cross and moved from side to side, the cross that is seen moves *against* the direction of movement. Using a concave lens, the cross that is seen moves *with* the direction of movement. When a toric lens is used, the cross that is seen is distorted and 'scissors' as the lens is moved. A prismatic lens cannot be centred over both arms of the cross since it has no optical centre, so one arm of the cross is always displaced with respect to the other. A Geneva lens measure is calibrated for crown glass lenses.[1]

**Difficulty level: 3**

**47**   i. F      ii. T      iii. T      iv. F      v. F

The duochrome test is based on the principle of ocular chromatic aberration, where short wavelengths are deviated more on refraction than long wavelengths. The test is able to detect an alteration in refraction of 0.25 dioptres or less. A myope sees the red letters more clearly and a hypermetrope sees the green letters more clearly. At the end of subjective refraction, a myope should be left seeing the red letters slightly better (i.e. slightly undercorrected), as if they are left hypermetropic the patient will need to accommodate for distance vision. The test can be used in colour-blind patients, since one set of letters will still appear clearer than the other depending on their refraction.[1]

**Difficulty level: 3**

**48**   i. T     ii. T     iii. F     iv. T     v. T

Oblique astigmatism occurs when incident light strikes a spherical lens at an angle that is not parallel to the principal axis of the lens. This introduces a toric effect. Oblique astigmatism is more problematic in biconvex or biconcave lenses. In most daily activities, an adult's line of vision is slightly below the principal axis of a spectacle lens, and so most lenses are slightly tilted (pantoscopic tilt) to account for this and minimise oblique astigmatism.

The eye reduces oblique astigmatism by the aplanatic nature of the cornea, and also since the retina is curved, the circle of least confusion formed by the induced toric effect still falls on the retina.[1]

**Difficulty level: 3**

**49**   i. T     ii. F     iii. F     iv. T     v. F

Axial hypermetropia results when the eye is too short for its refractive power. Refractive hypermetropia is when the refractive power of the eye is not adequate (e.g. in aphakia).

Manifest hypermetropia is the strongest convex lens correction that can be accepted for clear distance vision.

Latent hypermetropia is the residual hypermetropia which is involuntarily corrected for by ciliary tone and accommodation.

Facultative hypermetropia is that which can be overcome by accommodation.

Absolute hypermetropia is that which cannot be overcome by maximum accommodation.[1]

**Difficulty level: 3**

**50**   i. F     ii. T     iii. T     iv. F     v. F

This person has 3 dioptres of accommodation remaining but to read comfortably should keep one third of this in reserve, i.e. 2 dioptres can be used. To read at 25 cm (0.25 m), 4 dioptres accommodation are required, i.e. 1/0.25. Therefore the presbyopic correction required is the difference between these values, i.e. 2 dioptres. To read at 20 cm, 5 dioptres (i.e. 1/0.2) of accommodation are required. Since 2 dioptres of the patient's own accommodation is used, a 3-dioptre presbyopic correction is required.[1]

**Difficulty level: 3**

**51**  i. F  ii. T  iii. T  iv. F  v. T

The retinal cones are more sensitive to light that enters the eye paraxially than that which enters obliquely. This (the Stiles-Crawford effect) helps to reduce spherical aberration in the eye. Since cones are affected, photopic vision is affected more than scotopic vision. The troland is a measure of illumination when one candela per square metre is viewed through a pupil entrance of one square millimetre after correction for the Stiles-Crawford effect.[1]
   **Difficulty level: 3**

**52**  i. T  ii. F  iii. T  iv. F  v. T

Spectacle correction of aphakia causes magnification of the image, with a magnification effect of 1.33. Therefore, objects appear nearer than they are, and Snellen visual acuity testing may be enhanced due to the larger image seen. The high-powered lenses are heavy and so may slip down the patient's nose, increasing their effectivity. Spherical aberration causes image distortion (pincushion effect) when light does not pass through the axial zone of the lens.[1]
   **Difficulty level: 3**

**53**  i. F  ii. F  iii. F  iv. T  v. F

The SRK formula states:

Lens power = A constant − (2.5 × axial length) − (0.9 × average K readings)

Therefore, 118 − (2.5 × 22.1) − (0.9 × 43) = 24.05 dioptres.[1]
   **Difficulty level: 3**

**54**  i. T  ii. F  iii. F  iv. T  v. F

In 'with the rule' astigmatism, the steeper corneal meridian (i.e. the more powerful one) is closer to 90 degrees. In 'against the rule' the steeper corneal meridian is closer to 180 degrees.
   A corneal incision 'weakens' the cornea in that meridian. Therefore, in a patient that has 'with the rule' astigmatism, a superior corneal incision would reduce the power in the steeper meridian and reduce the astigmatism. A temporal incision would further reduce the power in the weaker meridian and worsen the astigmatism. Limbal relaxing incisions or more rarely arcuate keratotomy centred on the 90-degree meridian may be used in addition to reduce 'with the rule' astigmatism at the time of cataract surgery. A toric lens

with negative power in the 90-degree meridian would be needed to correct 'with the rule' astigmatism.[2]

**Difficulty level: 3**

**55**    i. T      ii. T      iii. F      iv. F      v. F

The Farnsworth-Munsell test comprises 84 coloured discs in four groups. Each disc varies in hue but brightness and saturation are equal. The discs in each group must be arranged in order of colour. The D-15 test uses colours from all parts of the spectrum that have to be arranged in order from a reference colour. The Ishihara test plates specifically test red-green defects. The VISITECH chart is a test of contrast sensitivity and the Vernier acuity test examines visual acuity.[1]

**Difficulty level: 4**

**56**    i. T      ii. T      iii. F      iv. T      v. T

A convex lens converges incident light parallel to the principal axis of the lens, and therefore has a positive vergence power.

Lens power = $1/f_2$

Where $f_2$ is the second focal length in metres, therefore an 8-dioptre lens has a 12.5-cm focal length.

A convex lens magnifies an image placed at or inside its first principal focus, therefore convex lenses are used in magnifying loupes.

Prismatic power = $F \times D$

where F is lens power in dioptres and D is decentration in centimetres.[1]

**Difficulty level: 2**

**57**    i. F      ii. F      iii. T      iv. F      v. F

Regarding retinoscopy reflexes, if a 'with movement' is seen, further convex lenses must be added and if an 'against movement' is seen, further concave lenses must be added. If the reflex moves obliquely off axis, astigmatism has not been neutralised. When one meridian has been neutralised, the reflex will align with the axis of the cylindrical lens and move with the direction of the retinoscopy streak. A scissor reflex can be seen near the endpoint of retinoscopy where one area is still relatively myopic and the other hypermetropic. A swirling reflex is a sign of keratoconus.[1]

**Difficulty level: 4**

**58**   i. F   ii. F   iii. T   iv. F   v. F

With the Maddox rod, the two eyes see different images and so a latent squint can become manifest. The right eye sees a line and the left eye the point source of light. The eye deviates in the opposite direction to where the red line is seen, therefore in this case the patient has an esophoria.[1]

**Difficulty level: 4**

**59**   i. T   ii. F   iii. T   iv. F   v. F

When an object is placed outside the first principal focus of a convex lens, the image formed is real, inverted and outside the second principal focus.[1]

**Difficulty level: 3**

**60**   i. F   ii. F   iii. T   iv. T   v. F

Unilateral spectacle magnification of aphakia results in an image that is magnified by one-third with respect to the other eye. Aniseikonia (the difference in size of the perceived images between the two eyes) may result, leading to the inability to fuse the images and therefore diplopia.[1]

**Difficulty level: 3**

## References

1  Elkington AR, Frank HJ, Greaney MJ. *Clinical Optics*. 3rd ed. Oxford: Blackwell Publishing; 2006. (**q31**) pp. 155–6, (**q32, q33**) pp. 162–3, (**q34**) pp. 244–9, (**q35**) pp. 253–4, (**q36**) p. 2, (**q37**) pp. 5, 17–18, (**q38**) pp. 30–1, (**q39**) pp. 36–7, (**q40**) pp. 45–6, (**q41**) pp. 49–52, (**q42**) p. 59, (**q43**) pp. 64–5, (**q44**) pp. 67–9, (**q45**) pp. 70–1, (**q46**) pp. 79–82, (**q47**) pp. 91–2, (**q48**) pp. 95–6, (**q49**) p. 114, (**q50**) p. 142, (**q51**) p. 94, (**q52**) pp. 130–1, (**q53**) p. 136, (**q55**) pp. 3, 4, 15, 16, (**q56**) pp. 57–64, (**q57**) pp. 232–5, (**q58**) p. 69, (**q59**) p. 58, (**q60**) p. 133.
2  Keirl A, Christie C. *Clinical Optics and Refraction*. 1st ed. Philadelphia: Balliere Tindall, Elsevier; 2007. (**q54**) p. 58.

# 8. Therapeutics FRCOphth answers

1 **A**  An ointment prolongs contact time with the cornea, increasing ocular penetration. The corneal epithelium is very permeable to fat-soluble molecules, so lipophilic drugs have higher permeability than hydrophilic drugs which permeate this layer poorly. (However, the stroma is hydrophilic and so drugs must also be water soluble to some extent.) Reflex tearing washes the drug out of the conjunctival sac. Administering multiple drops does not increase availability of the drug, but may cause systemic toxicity.[1]
**Difficulty level: 3**

2 **D**  Tissue binding such as melanin binding atropine leaves the drug unavailable and lengthens its presence in the compartment. Therefore, its efficacy is reduced but its action is prolonged.

First-order kinetics is where elimination is directly proportional to drug concentration, and therefore drug concentration decays exponentially. Zero-order kinetics is where drug elimination is at a constant rate and independent of concentration, i.e. it is linear.

Active transport is the movement of a substance usually across a cell membrane, in conjunction with the expenditure of energy such as ATP or creating an electrochemical gradient.[2]
**Difficulty level: 3**

3 **A**  The quinolones such as ciprofloxacin show better penetration into the eye than other antibiotic classes. Laevofloxacin and ofloxacin may have even better penetration than ciprofloxacin.[3]
**Difficulty level: 3**

4 **B**  In the eye, α receptors are present in dilator pupillae and Müller's muscle. Thus their stimulation causes pupil dilation and Müller's muscle acts with levator palpebrae superioris to elevate the eyelid. They are also present in conjunctival blood vessels and stimulation (such as with phenylephrine) causes their constriction and blanching of the conjunctiva.[4]
**Difficulty level: 3**

5 **A**  There are four main types of adrenergic receptor: stimulation of α1 receptors leads to smooth muscle contraction. Alpha-2 (α2) receptors are present on presynaptic neurons and are inhibitory. Beta-1 (β1) receptors are present in the heart and stimulation leads to increased force of contraction and heart rate, and also raises blood pressure. Hypotension

and bradycardia result from β1 receptor blockade. Beta-2 (β2) receptor stimulation causes smooth muscle relaxation in bronchi and blood vessels. Therefore, beta blockade causes constriction of smooth muscle in bronchial walls and can precipitate asthma. Beta blockers reduce aqueous secretion and therefore lower intraocular pressure.[4]
**Difficulty level: 3**

6   C   Apraclonidine is a relatively selective α2 agonist which does not cross the blood-brain barrier so has few side effects. It may cause a dry mouth and nose, in addition to conjunctival blanching. It is not used for prolonged periods due to tachyphylaxis resulting from the downregulation of receptors.[5]
**Difficulty level: 3**

7   C   Pilocarpine is a direct agonist of muscarinic acetylcholine receptor (a G-protein coupled receptor) and may be used topically to reduce intraocular pressure. It causes miosis and will reverse mydriasis caused by atropine but not that due to phenylephrine. It also causes contraction of the ciliary muscle leading to relaxation of the zonules and thickening of the lens and may result in accommodative spasm, which is especially symptomatic in young people. Ciliary muscle contraction and/or the anterior displacement of the iris-lens diaphragm may raise traction on the peripheral retina, and so is associated with increased risk of retinal tears.[5]
**Difficulty level: 4**

8   D   Accommodation is impaired by parasympathetic antagonists which act on the ciliary body. Phenylephrine is an adrenergic alpha receptor agonist and causes mydriasis without inhibiting accommodation.[5]
**Difficulty level: 3**

9   B   Acetazolamide is a carbonic anhydrase inhibitor and is derived from sulphonamides (as is sulphasalazine) so should not be given to patients with sulphonamide allergy.

Carbonic anhydrase catalyses the reversible reaction $H^+ + HCO_3^- \leftrightarrow H_2CO_3$, and in the non-pigmented ciliary epithelium, stimulates aqueous production by increasing availability of bicarbonate ions. Thus blocking this enzyme with acetazolamide may cause a metabolic acidosis. Acetazolamide may cause a transient myopia, probably related to reduced aqueous production and shallowing of the anterior chamber.[5]
**Difficulty level: 4**

**10 C** Mannitol is an osmotic agent (along with glycerol) that acts by increasing plasma osmotic pressure relative to aqueous and vitreous, thus drawing water out of these structures and reducing intraocular pressure. It is not absorbed by the GI tract so cannot be given orally. Mannitol is not metabolised significantly so is safe to use in diabetics, whereas glycerol is metabolised to glucose. The fluid shifts associated with hyperosmotic agents may cause congestive cardiac failure, pulmonary oedema or renal failure, and so should be avoided or used with extreme caution in patients with a history of these conditions.[6]
**Difficulty level: 2**

**11 C** Latanoprost is a prostaglandin F2α derivative and acts on FP prostanoid receptors in the eye. It reduces intraocular pressure by reducing uveoscleral outflow and has little effect on aqueous production. Latanoprost is generally safe to use in patients with asthma; caution should be taken in using beta blockers in asthmatic patients. Side effects include darkening of iris colour due to increased melanogenesis, growth of eyelashes and hyperaemia (usually mild). There are also reports of increased cystoid macular oedema with topical latanoprost use.[5]
**Difficulty level: 3**

**12 C** There are four classes of histamine receptor: $H_1$, $H_2$, $H_3$ and $H_4$, of which $H_1$ and $H_2$ receptors are the best-characterised ones. Stimulation of $H_1$ receptors causes contraction of smooth muscle in the ileum, bronchi and uterus. It also causes blood vessel dilation and increased heart rate and output. $H_2$ receptor stimulation causes increased gastric acid secretion.

$H_2$ blockers such as ranitidine act to reduce gastric acid production. Answers a, b and d are caused by histamine itself.[2]
**Difficulty level: 3**

**13 B** Steroids are lipid soluble so can permeate the cell membrane and bind to intracellular receptors. The steroid-receptor complex then travels to the nucleus where it acts by altering DNA transcription.[7]
**Difficulty level: 4**

**14 A** The majority of non-steroidal anti-inflammatory drugs (NSAIDs) act by inhibiting the enzyme cyclooxygenase (COX), leading to reduced prostaglandin synthesis. They also have free radical scavenging activity. There are two COX enzymes: COX-1 is present in most tissues and COX-2 in inflammatory cells. In recent years, increased risk of vascular thrombotic

events has been reported with COX-2 inhibitors and high-dose traditional NSAIDs.[2,8]
**Difficulty level: 4**

**15 B** 5-Fluorouracil is a pyrimidine analogue that leads to inhibition of DNA synthesis. It acts on highly proliferating cells in the mitotic phase of the cell cycle, and in the eye inhibits fibroblast proliferation and fibrosis. It has multiple uses, including as an adjunct in glaucoma surgery, reducing the risk of bleb failure postoperatively and also in pterygium surgery.[9]
**Difficulty level: 4**

**16 B** Cyclosporin A is a calcineurin inhibitor and has a relatively selective action on T-lymphocytes. It is metabolised by the P450 system in the liver, and has dose-dependent nephrotoxicity. It may cause gum hyperplasia.[2]
**Difficulty level: 4**

**17 C** Lignocaine is a short-acting local anaesthetic with rapid onset whose action lasts for approximately 2 hours. The mechanism of action is by preventing voltage-dependent sodium ion influx across axonal membranes, which in turn blocks the initiation and propagation of an action potential. Lignocaine is a weak base and is mainly metabolised in the liver.[2]
**Difficulty level: 3**

**18 B** Suxamethonium is a depolarising blocker of the neuromuscular junction, and thus is an agonist at post-synaptic acetylcholine receptors. It is not reversed by anticholinesterase drugs (unlike non-depolarising blockers). Suxamethonium may cause transient release of potassium from muscle fibres, leading to hyperkalaemia. It may cause raised intraocular pressure due to causing contraction of extraocular muscles which then place pressure on the globe.[2]
**Difficulty level: 4**

**19 B** Botulinum toxin is a highly potent bacterial exotoxin produced by the anaerobic bacterium *Clostridium botulinum*. There are eight serotypes of botulinum toxin of which serotypes A and less commonly B are used clinically. It prevents release of acetylcholine from nerve terminals. It can be used to induce a temporary ptosis to protect the corneal epithelium in cases of corneal ulceration or exposure. It can also be used to treat blepharospasm, and in the management of squint.[2]
**Difficulty level: 4**

**20 D** Ethambutol, amiodarone and vigabatrin may cause an optic neuropathy. Steroids are associated with cataract, increased intraocular pressure and increased risk of developing idiopathic intracranial hypertension.[10]
**Difficulty level: 3**

## References

1 Urtti A. Challenges and obstacles of ocular pharmacokinetics and drug delivery. *Adv Drug Deliver Rev.* 2006; **58**(11): 1131–5 **(q1)**.

2 Rang HP, Dale MM, Ritter JM, *et al. Rang and Dale's Pharmacology.* 7th ed. Philadelphia: Churchill Livingstone Elsevier; 2011. **(q2)** pp. 125–9 **(q12)** p. 211, **(q14)** p. 318, **(q16)** pp. 328–9, **(q17)** pp. 525–9, **(q18)** p. 166, **(q19)** pp. 167–8.

3 Cantor LB, Wuunn D, Yung CW, *et al.* Ocular penetration of levofloxacin, ofloxacin and ciprofloxacin in eyes with functioning filtering blebs: investigator masked, randomised clinical trial. *Br J Ophthalmol.* 2008; **92**: 345–7 **(q3)**.

4 Forrester J, Dick A, McMenamin A, *et al. The Eye: basic sciences in practice.* 2nd ed. Philadelphia: Saunders Elsevier; 2007. **(q4, q5)** p. 284.

5 Bartlett, JD, Jaanus SD. *Clinical Ocular Pharmacology.* Oxford: Butterworth Heinemann Elsevier; 2008. **(q6)** p. 155, **(q7)** pp. 168–70, **(q8)** p. 345, **(q9)** p. 162, **(q11)** pp. 139–43.

6 Schacknow PN, Samples JR. *The Glaucoma Book: a practical, evidence-based approach to patient care.* New York: Springer; 2010. **(q10)** p. 612.

7 Alberts B, Johnson A, Lewis J, *et al. Molecular Biology of the Cell.* 4th ed. New York: Garland Science; 2002. Chapter 15 **(q13)**.

8 Kearney PM, Baigent C, Godwin J, *et al.* Do selective cyclo-oxygenase-2 inhibitors and traditional non-steroidal anti-inflammatory drugs increase the risk of atherothrombosis? Meta-analysis of randomised trials. *BMJ.* 2006; **332**: 1302–8 **(q14)**.

9 Abraham LM, Selva D, Casson R, *et al.* The clinical applications of fluorouracil in ophthalmic practice. *Drugs.* 2007; **67**(2): 237–55 **(q15)**.

10 Kanski JJ. *Clinical Ophthalmology – a systematic approach.* 6th ed. Edinburgh: Butterworth Heinemann Elsevier; 2007. **(q20)** p. 840.

# 8. Therapeutics ICO answers

**21**   i. F      ii. F      iii. T      iv. T      v. T

Drug antagonism occurs when the effect of one drug is reduced or blocked by another. There are several types of drug antagonism, which include:

a) Pharmacokinetic antagonism when one drug affects the absorption, metabolism or excretion of another; for example, sulphonylureas inducing liver enzymes and increasing warfarin metabolism, which therefore decreases warfarin levels.
b) Competitive antagonism occurs when both drugs bind to the same receptor. It can be reversible if increasing the concentration of the agonist overcomes the antagonist. It is irreversible if the antagonist dissociates very slowly or not at all from drug receptors, so cannot be overcome by increasing the agonist dose.
c) Non-competitive antagonism where the antagonist acts downstream of the receptor to block some part of the pathway involved in producing a response.
d) Physiological antagonism in which two drugs with opposing actions in the body cancel each other out.[1]
**Difficulty level: 4**

**22**   i. T      ii. F      iii. F      iv. F      v. T

G-proteins mediate the interaction between a receptor and the target protein. G-proteins are membrane bound and consist of three subunits: the alpha subunit which is a GTPase that catalyses conversion of GTP to GDP, and the beta and gamma subunits which anchor the protein into the plasma membrane. When the G-protein binds to an agonist-bound receptor, the alpha subunit dissociates which is then able to interact with a target protein.

Binding of an agonist molecule to a G-protein coupled receptor can activate several G-protein molecules, which may amplify the signal.

Muscarinic acetylcholine receptors and beta-adrenoreceptors are examples of G-protein coupled receptors.[1]
**Difficulty level: 4**

**23**   i. F   ii. F   iii. F   iv. T   v. T

Common methods of local anaesthesia for cataract surgery include topical anaesthesia (with or without intracameral anaesthesia), sub-Tenon's anaesthesia, peribulbar (i.e. extraconal) anaesthesia and retrobulbar (intraconal) anaesthesia. The latter is rarely used. Globe and conjunctival anaesthesia are achieved by blockade of the ophthalmic and maxillary branches of the trigeminal nerve. Akinesia is achieved by blockade of the ophthalmic parts of cranial nerves III, IV and VI. All methods of delivery of anaesthesia except topical also cause akinesia. High doses of topical anaesthesia may cause corneal erosion due to epithelial toxicity. Peribulbar block may cause proptosis.[2]

**Difficulty level: 3**

**24**   i. F   ii. T   iii. T   iv. F   v. T

Azathioprine is an immunosuppressant drug. It is metabolised to 6-mercaptopurine, which inhibits purine synthesis. The major side effects incurred include bone marrow suppression and hepatotoxicity, therefore full blood count and liver function tests must be regularly monitored. 6-mercaptopurine is metabolised by the enzyme thiopurine S-methyltransferase (TPMT) and polymorphisms in this enzyme may lead to azathioprine toxicity. Therefore, many centres check serum TPMT levels prior to commencing therapy.[1]

**Difficulty level: 4**

**25**   i. F   ii. F   iii. F   iv. T   v. T

Brimonidine is an $\alpha2$ agonist. It is less effective than latanoprost, but is useful in further reducing intraocular pressure in patients that are uncontrolled on latanoprost. Brimonidine causes miosis especially under scotopic conditions and so may be useful in treating glare in patients who have had refractive surgery. The main ocular side effects are hyperaemia, burning and stinging. Systemic effects include dry mouth, headache and fatigue.[3]

**Difficulty level: 3**

**26**   i. F   ii. T   iii. F   iv. F   v. T

Tachyphylaxis is a decreased response to a drug, or decreased effectiveness with repeated exposure. It is frequently seen with long-term apraclonidine therapy. Beta-blocker therapy also shows a longer-term reduction in responsiveness, with reports suggesting less than half the eyes initially treated with beta blockers are on the original therapy alone at five years.[3]

**Difficulty level: 3**

27    i.   F      ii.   F      iii.   T      iv.   T      v.   T

Dorzolamide is a topical carbonic anhydrase inhibitor and acts via inhibiting aqueous production. Since it is a sulphonamide derivative, it is relatively contraindicated in patients with sulphonamide allergy. Local side effects include an ocular burning sensation, allergic conjunctivitis and periorbital contact dermatitis, which resolves on cessation of treatment. It may leave a bitter taste in the mouth after administration.[4]

**Difficulty level: 3**

28    i.   F      ii.   F      iii.   T      iv.   F      v.   T

Adverse effects due to oral antihistamines, especially first-generation drugs, include palpitations, dry eyes and mouth, gastrointestinal tract disturbances and urinary frequency. However, due to blockade of muscarinic acetylcholine, serotonin and alpha adrenergic receptors, other effects such as mydriasis and urinary retention also occur. The first-generation drugs may cause significant drowsiness; however, due to reduced lipid solubility, the second-generation antihistamines such as cetirizine penetrate the central nervous system less, resulting in little sedative effect.[3]

**Difficulty level: 3**

29    i.   T      ii.   F      iii.   F      iv.   F      v.   F

Benzalkonium chloride (BAK) is a commonly used preservative in eye drops. It is bactericidal and attaches to the bacterial cell wall, increasing its permeability. BAK is most effective at approximately pH 8 and is inactivated in the presence of salts such as magnesium and calcium. Many solutions therefore also contain EDTA to chelate these ions. It may cause direct toxicity to the cornea or a hypersensitivity reaction such as conjunctivitis, keratitis and corneal oedema.[5]

**Difficulty level: 4**

**30**    i. T        ii. T        iii. F        iv. T        v. T

Chloroquine is toxic to the retina in a dose-dependent manner: the risk of toxicity is high when the cumulative dose exceeds 300 g. Hydroxychloroquine is much safer and there is little risk of retinopathy if the dose is below 400 mg per day.[6]

**Difficulty level: 2**

**31**    i. F        ii. T        iii. F        iv. T        v. T

Topical steroids are most commonly associated with the development of posterior subcapsular cataract. Raised intraocular pressure is a known side effect and is more common in patients known to have open angle glaucoma or a family history of glaucoma, diabetes mellitus or high myopia. The mechanism of action is not clear but may involve activation of steroid receptors on the trabecular meshwork altering expression of trabecular meshwork genes. Another theory is that steroids cause accumulation of glycosaminoglycans in the trabecular meshwork. Steroids may also cause central serous retinopathy and thinning of the sclera, the latter with chronic use.[7]

**Difficulty level: 3**

**32**    i. T        ii. F        iii. T        iv. T        v. F

Ligand-gated ion channels are transmembrane proteins containing a central aqueous channel. Following ligand binding the channels open rapidly, and therefore these receptors are involved mainly in fast synaptic transmission and in the generation of action potentials. Nicotinic acetylcholine, GABA A and $5HT_3$ receptors are examples.[1]

**Difficulty level: 4**

**33**    i. T        ii. T        iii. F        iv. F        v. F

Many drugs undergo enzymatic modification in their metabolism. Phase I reactions involve oxidation, reduction or hydrolysis and often involve the P450 enzyme system in the liver. Phase II reactions involve conjugation. Drugs such as rifampicin that induce liver enzymes cause increased metabolism. First-pass metabolism involves a significant reduction of drug concentration before it reaches the systemic circulation, usually due to removal from the portal circulation by liver metabolism or metabolism in the wall of the intestine.[1]

**Difficulty level: 4**

**34**   i. T      ii. T      iii. T      iv. T      v. T

Dyspepsia is one of the commonest side effects, and inhibition of prostaglandin $E_2$, which is protective to the gastric mucosa, may cause ulceration. Prostaglandins are also involved in maintaining renal blood flow dynamics, so their inhibition may precipitate acute renal failure. Hepatitis and bone marrow suppression may occur but are rare.[1,8]
   **Difficulty level: 3**


**35**   i. T      ii. T      iii. T      iv. F      v. F

Thiopurine S-methyltransferase (TPMT) polymorphisms may affect azathioprine metabolism. N-acetyltransferase deficiency affects isoniazid metabolism. Dapsone metabolism may be significantly affected in patients with glucose-6-phosphate dehydrogenase (G6PD) deficiency.[9]
   **Difficulty level: 4**


**36**   i. F      ii. T      iii. T      iv. F      v. F

For treatment of endophthalmitis, intraocular vancomycin is generally considered to be the drug of choice for treating Gram-positive organisms. For Gram-negative organisms, amikacin or ceftazidime may be used. Aminoglycosides such as gentamicin may cause retinal toxicity when injected intravitreally.[10]
   **Difficulty level: 4**


**37**   i. T      ii. T      iii. F      iv. F      v. F

Drugs that are able to saturate metabolizing liver enzymes may show zero-order kinetics. This means drug elimination is at a constant rate and independent of concentration, i.e. it is linear. Examples are aspirin and phenytoin.[1]
   **Difficulty level: 5**


**38**   i. F      ii. F      iii. T      iv. T      v. T

Methotrexate is a folate antagonist and acts via inhibition of dihydrofolate reductase. It is used in the treatment of scleritis and uveitis often as a steroid-sparing agent. It is excreted by the kidney. Side effects include bone marrow depression, raised liver function tests, oral ulceration, myalgia and pneumonitis.[1,11]
   **Difficulty level: 3**

**39**   i. F      ii. F      iii. F      iv. T      v. T

Opioids are potent analgesics and act via μ-, δ-, κ- and σ-receptors which are G-protein coupled. Pupil constriction is a centrally mediated effect due to stimulation of receptors in the oculomotor nucleus. Opiates may also cause respiratory depression, constipation, pruritus, cough suppression, broncho-constriction and sedation.[1]
**Difficulty level: 4**

**40**   i. T      ii. T      iii. F      iv. F      v. T

Acetazolamide is a carbonic anhydrase inhibitor and reduces intraocular pressure via reduction of aqueous production. It may also be used to treat cystoid macular oedema and idiopathic intracranial hypertension. Side effects include paraesthesia, metallic taste, fatigue and nausea. Inhibition of carbonic anhydrase in the renal proximal tubule leads to reduced bicarbonate absorption and metabolic alkalosis. Acetazolamide may also cause thrombocytopaenia, agranulocytosis and aplastic anaemia.[3]
**Difficulty level: 3**

# References

1  Rang HP, Dale MM, Ritter JM, *et al. Rang and Dale's Pharmacology*. 7th ed. Philadelphia: Churchill Livingstone Elsevier; 2011. (**q21**) p. 15, (**q22**) p. 31, (**q24**) p. 330, (**q32**) pp. 26–7, (**q33**) pp. 115–18, (**q34**) pp. 321–3, (**q37**) p. 128, (**q38**) p. 327, (**q39**) pp. 514–5.

2  Malik A, Fletcher EC, Chong V, *et al.* Local anaesthesia for cataract surgery. *JCRS.* 2010; **36**: 133–52 (**q23**).

3  Bartlett, JD, Jaanus SD. *Clinical Ocular Pharmacology*. Oxford. Butterworth Heinemann Elsevier; 2008. (**q25**) p. 157, (**q26**) pp. 145, 154, (**q28**) pp. 250–3, (**q40**) p. 162.

4  Shaarawy T, Sherwood M, Hitchings R, *et al. Glaucoma Volume One: Medical Diagnosis & Therapy*. Philadelphia: Saunders Elsevier; 2009. (**q27**) p. 543.

5  Forrester J, Dick A, McMenamin A, *et al. The Eye: basic sciences in practice*. 2nd ed. Philadelphia: Saunders Elsevier; 2007. (**q29**) p. 280.

6  Kanski JJ. *Clinical Ophthalmology – a systematic approach*. 6th ed. Edinburgh: Butterworth Heinemann Elsevier; 2007. (**q30**) p. 840.

7  Carnahan MC, Goldstein DA. Ocular complications of topical, peri-ocular, and systemic corticosteroids. *Curr Opin Ophthalmol.* 2000; **11**: 478–83 (**q31**).

8  Kearney PM, Baigent C, Godwin J, *et al.* Do selective cyclo-oxygenase-2 inhibitors and traditional non-steroidal anti-inflammatory drugs increase the risk of

atherothrombosis? Meta-analysis of randomised trials. *BMJ*. 2006; **332**: 1302–8 (**q34**).

9  Shenfield GM. Genetic polymorphisms, drug metabolism and drug concentrations. *Clin Biochem Rev*. 2004; **25**(4): 203–6 (**q35**).

10  Roth DB, Flynn HW. Antibiotic selection in the treatment of endophthalmitis: the significance of drug combinations and synergy. *Surv Ophthalmol*. 1997; **41**(5): 395–401 (**q36**).

11  Huang JJ, Gaudio PA. *Ocular Inflammatory Disease and Uveitis Manual: diagnosis & treatment*. Philadelphia: Lippincott Williams & Wilkins; 2010. (**q38**) p. 220.

# 9. Lasers and instruments FRCOphth answers

1  **A**  Wavelengths of 400–1400 µm penetrate the eye.[1]
**Difficulty level: 2**

2  **A**  White light is emitted by the camera, passing through a blue 'excitation' filter to illuminate the fundus with blue light. The blue reflected light and yellow-green fluorescent light leaving the eye are separated by a yellow-green barrier filter in the camera. This blocks blue light and exposes the camera to yellow-green from the fluorescein.[2]
**Difficulty level: 2**

3  **A**  Holmium lasers are used to create sclerostomies, and thereby increase aqueous humour outflow. Nd-YAG laser is typically used to disrupt the posterior capsule. Diode lasers are absorbed by melanin, whereas argon blue-green laser is absorbed by melanin *and* haemoglobin.[1]
**Difficulty level: 3**

4  **B**  The red-free filter on the slit-lamp helps visualise structures stained with Rose Bengal. Blue cobalt is the best filter for visualising fluorescein staining.[2]
**Difficulty level: 2**

5  **B**  The direct ophthalmoscope consists of lenses which focus an electric light onto a mirror. The mirror reflects the light which is used to illuminate the patient's eye. In order to maximise the field of view it is important

to be as close as possible to the patient's eye. Light is reflected back through the hole in the mirror and into the observer's eye. If the dioptric power of the eye is +60 D, then using the loupe formula M = F/4 where M is the magnification and F the dioptric power of the loupe, this gives the magnification as x15.[2]

**Difficulty level: 2**

6  C  Surgical lasers are capable of damaging the eye and are classified as 3b or 4. Therefore strict safety regulations, such as the use of protective filters and goggles, must be adhered to.[1]

**Difficulty level: 4**

7  C  Energy is usually delivered to atoms in a laser active medium, allowing atoms to move from their ground state to a higher energy level. Atoms at this 'excited state' are unstable and emit light energy.[1]

**Difficulty level: 4**

8  C  The image formed will be between the condensing lens and the observer, and will be a real image that is *both* vertically and laterally inverted. It is focused to a point between the examiner and the lens.[2]

**Difficulty level: 3**

9  D  Q-switching creates a brief pulse rather than a continuous wave of laser. The energy output of a laser depends on the shutter speed used. Q-switching is a mechanism whereby a shutter is placed in front of one of the two mirrors in the laser tube. This maximises the energy state of the laser medium by limiting energy loss to spontaneous emission alone.[1]

**Difficulty level: 4**

10 A  Scanning laser polarimetry uses the principle of birefringence. Polarised light passes through nerve fibre layer, after which it is partially reflected back through the nerve fibre layer and this induces an alteration in the polarisation of light. The size of this is known as retardation.

Confocal scanning laser tomography uses a diode laser and produces an image of the optic nerve head. The initial image is taken in the retinal plane and subsequent images are taken with the focal plane moved posteriorly towards the lamina cribrosa.

Laser interferometry projects two light sources on the retina, creating a sine wave grating. It allows the estimation of visual acuity when the macula cannot be seen.[1]

Confocal microscopy obtains detailed images of the cornea.

**Difficulty level: 4**

**11  B**  It is unlikely that the patient is 6.0D hypermetropic or myopic due to the uncorrected visual acuity. In addition accommodation is minimal at the age of 55. The most likely scenario is that the observer is accommodating to view the retina.[1]
**Difficulty level: 3**

**12  B**  The treatment of age-related macular degeneration (ARMD) with photodynamic therapy study (TAP) demonstrated that classic subfoveal ARMD lesions responded well. Recent advances in anti-VEGF therapies have superseded this treatment, although it is likely that there may be a role for combination therapy in years to come.[3]
**Difficulty level: 3**

**13  B**  Corneal pachymeters of the optical type use Purkinje-Sanson images I and II, which are formed by the anterior and posterior surfaces of the cornea. Images II and III are used to measure the depth of the anterior chamber.[1]
**Difficulty level: 4**

**14  C**  The microscope consists of two convex lenses. A real, inverted and magnified image is formed. Examples of a compound microscope are the slit-lamp and specular microscopes.[1]
**Difficulty level: 4**

**15  A**  The Javal-Schiotz keratometer is typically a two-positioned instrument which uses a fixed image and a doubling device to measure the radius of curvature of the cornea.[1]
**Difficulty level: 3**

**16  C**  A 20D lens is commonly used in indirect ophthalmoscopy.
A Koeppe lens is used for gonioscopy.
A Rodenstock lens is a high-positive contact lens. The entire fundus beyond the equator can be imaged.
A Hruby lens is a non-contact lens used for visualising the retina.
A Mainster lens is a contact lens used for visualising the retina.[1]
**Difficulty level: 3**

**17  D**  With a thicker cornea, greater applanation force is required to neutralise the surface rigidity of the cornea and therefore the intraocular pressure reading is likely to be artificially high. Corneal astigmatism will result in distorted mires, and 4 dioptres of astigmatism can elevate the intraocular pressure by 1 mmHg.[2]
**Difficulty level: 3**

18 **B**  A mean deviation is the mean of all of the deviations. A high value represents an overall depression from an age-matched control. This would be seen in cataract. A pattern deviation can be described as a 'standard deviation of the deviations', and upgrades a globally depressed field, thereby illustrating focal deficits such as those seen in glaucoma.[2]
**Difficulty level: 3**

19 **D**  Green light is used to reduce chromatic aberration.[1,2]
**Difficulty level: 3**

20 **A**  It measures the surface curvature of the lens. The total power is the sum of the surface powers of the lens. The instrument is calibrated for crown glass and therefore a correction must be added for lenses made of other materials.[1]
**Difficulty level: 4**

21 **C**  The latest generation of automated Goldmann perimeters also offer static perimetry tests.[1]
**Difficulty level: 4**

22 **C**  The Tono-Pen is hand-held and as it uses a different tip each time it can be reused. It is a relatively straightforward instrument to use.[2]
**Difficulty level: 3**

23 **A**  The reflex will move in the same direction, therefore the examiner can infer that more 'plus' is required to neutralise and therefore correct the hypermetropia.[1]
**Difficulty level: 3**

24 **D**  The indirect ophthalmoscope consists of a condensing lens, which is a powerful convex lens. The illuminating light beam passes through the condensing lens into the eye and is then refracted by the condensing lens. This creates a real image between the observer and the condensing lens. The observer's pupil influences the field of view, along with the aperture of the condensing lens. The patient's pupil size determines the field of illumination.[2]
**Difficulty level: 3**

25 **C**  Optical coherence tomography is an interferometric non-invasive imaging technique. Light from an infrared source (843 nm) is split into a reference beam, which is reflected off a mirror, and a sample beam, reflected

off the retina. The temporal differences are converted to a digital signal and viewed. OCT is commonly used to view macular microstructure.[1]
**Difficulty level: 5**

## References

1 Elkington AR, Frank HJ, Greaney MJ. *Clinical Optics*. 3rd ed. Oxford: Blackwell Publishing; 2003. (**q1**) pp. 1–4, (**q3**) pp. 225–8, (**q6**) pp. 228–30, (**q7**) pp. 222–6, (**q9**) pp. 220–5, (**q10**) pp. 224–30, (**q11**) pp. 165–73, (**q13**) pp. 111–12, (**q14**) pp. 195–7, (**q15**) pp. 191–4, (**q16**) pp. 173–4, 200–4, (**q19, q20**) p. 82, (**q21**) pp. 89–91, (**q23**) pp. 230–42, (**q25**) p. 209.

2 Madge S, Kersey J, Hawker M, *et al*. *Clinical Techniques in Ophthalmology*. Edinburgh: Churchill Livingstone; 2006. (**q2**) pp. 145–6, (**q4**) pp. 125–7, (**q5**) pp. 58–60, (**q8**) pp. 53–5, (**q17**) pp. 132–6, (**q18**) pp. 87–9, (**q19**) pp. 62–5, (**q22**) p. 136, (**q24**) pp. 53–7.

3 Brown DM, Michels M, Kaiser PK, *et al*. Verteporfin photodynamic therapy combined with intravitreal bevacizumab for neovascular age-related macular degeneration, *Ophthalmology*. 2009; **116**(4): 747–55 (**q12**).

# 9. Lasers and instruments ICO answers

**26**  i. T  ii. T  iii. F  iv. F  v. F

A stereoscopic view is possible with the indirect ophthalmoscope as this is a binocular instrument. This is unlike the direct ophthalmoscope, which is a monocular instrument. The eyepieces usually contain a +2D lens which relaxes the observer's accommodation reflex. The image is inverted and the field of view is dependent upon the refractive error of the patient. A higher-power condensing lens produces a smaller image but a larger field of view.[1]
**Difficulty level: 2**

**27**  i. F  ii. F  iii. F  iv. T  v. T

With a direct ophthalmoscope, the magnification is dependent upon the refractive error of the patient. It can correct for spherical error, so a user with a degree of astigmatism would be advised to keep their spectacles on.[1]
**Difficulty level: 2**

**28**   i. F       ii. F       iii. F       iv. T       v. F

Keratometry is a process to measure corneal curvature and axis, and commonly used instruments are the Helmholtz or Javal-Schiotz keratometers. These measure two readings at 90 degrees to each other.[1]
   **Difficulty level: 3**


**29**   i. F       ii. T       iii. T       iv. F       v. T

The focimeter is used to measure spectacle lens power with both manual and automatic machines in production. Presbyopic patients may be wearing bifocals, and the strength of the addition lens can be calculated by the difference between the near and distance segments. With prismatic correction, the image may not be centred when looking through the eyepiece. The patient may therefore have diplopia.[1]
   **Difficulty level: 3**


**30**   i. T       ii. F       iii. F       iv. T       v. F

Ninety-eight per cent of ICG molecules bind to proteins in the blood. The excitation peak for ICG is 805 nm, with emission at 815 nm. Indocyanine green should not be given to patients allergic to iodine, and pruritis is a common side effect.[2]
   **Difficulty level: 3**


**31**   i. F       ii. F       iii. T       iv. T       v. F

The Hruby lens is a high minus contact lens and can be used to visualise the retina. This produces an optically virtual but upright image. The panfundoscope and 28D lenses are used to examine the retina.[1]
   **Difficulty level: 2**


**32**   i. F       ii. T       iii. T       iv. T       v. T

Javal-Schiotz is the name of a keratometer rather than a tonometer.[1]
   **Difficulty level: 2**

**33**   i. T       ii. T       iii. F       iv. T       v. F

The Oculus Pentacam instrument is effective at measuring corneal thickness, both anterior and posterior curvature of the cornea and keratometric readings at a variety of radii from the central cornea. This makes it useful for monitoring in conditions such as keratoconus. Central corneal thickness is useful in glaucoma, and the information gathered is important for patients wishing to undergo corneal refractive surgery.[3]
   **Difficulty level: 3**

**34**   i. F       ii. T       iii. F       iv. T       v. F

Goldmann perimetry is useful in children and in the detection of neurological conditions that may affect the visual field. The patient is required to maintain gaze, and in this way the blind spot is mapped.[1]
   **Difficulty level: 3**

**35**   i. T       ii. F       iii. F       iv. F       v. T

Ishihara colour-vision testing was originally designed as a screening test for congenital red/green defects. It may be used for the testing of innumerate patients (13 plates are present at the back of the book containing patterns rather than numbers). Those with normal colour vision will see plates 10 and 17. The Farnsworth-Munsell 100-hue test can detect mild colour-vision abnormalities and consists of 84 movable tiles.[1]
   **Difficulty level: 4**

**36**   i. T       ii. F       iii. F       iv. F       v. T

Two Maddox rods may be used if a torsional phoria exists. This prism bar is also a useful instrument to use in this instance.[1]
   **Difficulty level: 4**

**37**   i. F       ii. F       iii. T       iv. F       v. F

The exophthalmometer is used to measure ocular protrusion. Reproducible measurements are often difficult with parallax being difficult to control. The feet of the exophthalmometer rest upon the lateral orbital rims.[1]
   **Difficulty level: 2**

**38**  i. F  ii. F  iii. F  iv. T  v. F

Laser light is, by and large, transverse within the laser tube and emitted in this way. Energy is delivered diffusely in argon laser photocoagulation, whereas it is delivered in a focused point for Nd-YAG capsulotomy. This achieves the greatest disruptive effect. When energy is focused on the smallest spot, this is known as the fundamental mode.[4]

**Difficulty level: 3**

**39**  i. T  ii. T  iii. F  iv. T  v. T

Lasers can have thermal, ionising, photodisruptive, audiological and scarring effects.[4]

**Difficulty level: 2**

**40**  i. T  ii. T  iii. F  iv. T  v. F

The argon laser is traditionally a mix of blue and green light. It treats the outer retina. Xanthophyll is blue light sensitive and therefore blue light lasers are not used at the macula as this will cause damage. A cataractous lens scatters the laser beam light and therefore a higher laser power is often used to produce the desired effect.[4]

**Difficulty level: 3**

**41**  i. T  ii. T  iii. F  iv. T  v. T

Lens pitting and corneal endothelial damage can occur when the laser is not focused properly.[1]

**Difficulty level: 2**

**42**  i. T  ii. T  iii. F  iv. F  v. F

The Nd-YAG laser is useful for capsulotomy following cataract surgery. The diode laser is useful for retinal or ciliary body ablation and the erbium: YAG laser has been used, only experimentally, for lens emulsification during cataract surgery.[4]

**Difficulty level: 4**

**43**  i. T      ii. T      iii. F      iv. F      v. T

The argon laser emits in the 480–510 nm wavelength range and the excimer emits in the ultraviolet range. The Holmium laser is a solid-state laser able to cut tissue in a liquid-filled environment (blood, saline) with the capability of fibre-optic delivery. It has exciting potential uses in ophthalmology as well as other fields such as urology and orthopaedics.[4,5]

**Difficulty level: 4**


**44**  i. F      ii. T      iii. T      iv. T      v. T

Anaphylaxis is a rare complication of intravenous fluorescein administration.[2]

**Difficulty level: 2**


**45**  i. F      ii. T      iii. T      iv. F      v. T

Royal College of Ophthalmology guidelines published in May 2008 state the use of transpupillary argon laser is the current gold standard in the treatment of retinopathy of prematurity. The recent emergence of anti-VEGF therapy may challenge this in the near future.[6,7]

**Difficulty level: 3**


**46**  i. T      ii. F      iii. T      iv. T      v. T

Thornton is a name applied to a fixation ring, used to steady the eye prior to incisions being made. Troutman is a name applied to a type of needle holder. A vectis is an instrument used to remove the lens in extracapsular cataract extraction. Apart from the vectis, the instruments are named after the ophthalmologists that invented them.[1]

**Difficulty level: 3**


**47**  i. T      ii. T      iii. F      iv. T      v. F

Nucleus expression in cataract surgery may be performed using a variety of instruments, including an irrigating vectis, viscoelastic and phacoemulsification. Viscoexpression and vectis use are usually part of an extracapsular cataract extraction technique.[8]

**Difficulty level: 3**

**48**   i. T      ii. F      iii. F      iv. F      v. T

Diode lasers emit energy with a wavelength of 810 nm, argon lasers between 480 and 510 nm, Nd-YAG lasers 1064 nm and excimer lasers between 180 and 210 nm.[4]

**Difficulty level: 3**

**49**   i. T      ii. F      iii. F      iv. T      v. T

This instrument utilises the retinal nerve fibre layer (RNFL) birefringence to correlate this with its thickness. The RNFL behaves as a birefringent medium as its axons are arranged in parallel. Light is reflected on the upper and lower layers. The birefringence of the RNFL changes the state of polarisation of light passing through it. The size of this change is known as retardation, and the amount of this correlates with the thickness of the layer.[4]

**Difficulty level: 4**

**50**   i. F      ii. F      iii. T      iv. T      v. T

Class 1 and 2 lasers tend to be safe for the human eye. Lasers used in ophthalmology tend to be classed as 3b or 4. CD players can be categorised as class 1 lasers, and laser pointers fall into the class 2 category.[4]

**Difficulty level: 4**

## References

1 Madge S, Kersey J, Hawker M, *et al*. *Clinical Techniques in Ophthalmology*. 1st ed. Edinburgh: Churchill Livingstone; 2006. (**q26**) pp. 53–5, (**q27**) pp. 58–9, (**q28**) pp. 66–7, (**q29**) pp. 63–6, (**q31**) pp. 128–30, (**q32**) pp. 138–40, (**q34**) pp. 90–1, (**q35**) pp. 82–3, (**q36**) pp. 36–7, (**q37**) pp. 72–3, (**q41**) pp. 210–12, (**q46**) pp. 202–5.

2 Kanski JJ. *Clinical Ophthalmology – a systematic approach*. 5th ed. Edinburgh: Butterworth Heinemann; 2003. (**q30**) pp. 397–401, (**q44**) pp. 395–400.

3 www.pentacam.com (**q33**) (accessed 4 April 2011)

4 Elkington AR, Frank HJ, Greaney MJ. *Clinical Optics*. 3rd ed. Oxford: Blackwell Publishing; 2006. (**q38**) pp. 218–20, (**q39**) pp. 218–22, (**q40**) p. 222–3, (**q42**) pp. 224–5, (**q43**) pp. 220–6, (**q48, q50**) pp. 228–30, (**q49**) pp. 226–8.

5 Holimum:YAG surgical lasers. *Health Devices*. 1995; **24**(3): 92–122 (**q43**).

6 Royal College of Ophthalmologists. *Guidelines for ROP screening*. May 2008. Available at: www.rcophth.ac.uk/page.asp?section=451&sectionTitle=Clinical+Guidelines (**q45**) (accessed 5 July 2011)

7 Mintz-Hitner H, Kennedy KA, Chuang AZ, *et al.* Efficacy of intravitreal bevacizumab for stage3+ retinopathy of prematurity. *N Engl J Med.* 2011; **364**(7): 603–14 (**q45**).

8 Bellucci R, Morselli S, Pucci V, *et al.* Nucleus viscoexpression compared with other techniques of nucleus removal in extracapsular cataract extraction with capsulorrhexis. *Ophthalmic Surg.* 1994; **25**(7): 432–7 (**q47**).

# 10. Epidemiology and biostatistics FRCOphth answers

**1 B** An outlier is an unusually high or low value in a data set – it can distort the mean, standard deviation and variance. Mean is the sum of the data values divided by the total number of values. The standard deviation is a statistical measure of the spread of a series of values. Variance is the square of the standard deviation. The median is the middle-most number when values are arranged from low to high. The median is not affected by outliers.[1]
**Difficulty level: 2**

**2 C** With a Gaussian (normal) distribution, 68.3% of data is within 1 standard deviation of the mean, 95.5% within 2 standard deviations and 99.8% within 3 standard deviations.[1]
**Difficulty level: 2**

**3 C** Group 1 entitlement (to drive motorcars and motorcycles) requires several criteria to be met. A person must have best corrected visual acuity in good light sufficient to read a vehicle registration plate where the characters are 50 mm wide at a distance of 20 metres. In practical terms, this equates to between the 6/9 and 6/12 line of a Snellen chart. In the presence of cataract, glare may prevent the vehicle registration plate being seen, even with apparently normal acuities. There should be no significant binocular field defect (defined as greater than 3 contiguous points missed) in at least 120 degrees on the horizontal scale and within 20 degrees above or below fixation on the vertical scale. New-onset diplopia is a contraindication to driving. Driving should cease until the diplopia is controlled with prisms or patching, the other driving visual requirements are met and

the patient has adapted – the DVLA can advise when driving can restart. Complete loss of vision in one eye is not a contraindication to driving a car provided the other eye has good visual acuity and full field, the driver has adapted to the deficit and the DVLA has been informed.[2]
**Difficulty level: 3**

4 **C** The visual standards for Group 2 entitlement (includes lorries and buses) are set higher. Best corrected visual acuity must be at least 6/9 in the better eye and no worse than 6/12 in the other eye. Uncorrected acuity in each eye must be at least 3/60. Glare from cataract should not prevent the above visual standards being met. Applicants with loss of vision in one eye or uncorrected acuity of less than 3/60 in one eye are barred in law from holding a Group 2 licence. A normal binocular field of vision is required. New-onset diplopia is a contraindication to driving. To regain a Group 2 licence the diplopia would have to be controlled with prisms and there would need to be suitable time for adaptation (patching would not be an option). Patients with colour blindness do not need to notify the DVLA.[2]
**Difficulty level: 3**

5 **B** The prevalence of visual impairment is extremely difficult to establish. In general, visual morbidity is under-reported. In developed countries, the prevalence of blindness is probably around 0.2%. The prevalence of blindness is much higher in developing countries, and in the least developed may be 3% or more.[3]
**Difficulty level: 4**

6 **B** Evidence from different study designs can be ranked in terms of hierarchy of evidence. The first rung is expert opinion, followed by case reports, then case series, case-control studies, cohort studies, randomised controlled double-masked trials and at the peak a meta-analysis of several peer-reviewed randomised double-masked controlled trials.[4]
**Difficulty level: 3**

7 **B** Patients are eligible for registration as severely sight impaired if best corrected visual acuity is less than 3/60, best corrected visual acuity is between 6/60 and 3/60 with field constriction, or best corrected visual acuity is greater than 6/60 (but not better than 6/18) with the field of vision severely constricted. Special recommendations apply with regard to the registration of young children.[5]
**Difficulty level: 3**

**8 C** The *p* value (significance level) is a measure of the probability that the results occurred by chance alone. With a *p* value of 0.05, if an experiment were carried out 100 times, the same result would occur 95 times and a different result 5 times because of chance.[1]
**Difficulty level: 2**

**9 D** A type I error occurs when one rejects the null hypothesis when in fact the results occurred by chance. A type II error occurs when one accepts the null hypothesis when in fact there really was a difference. Sampling error is bias of data based on choosing a non-representative sample of the population. The standard error is a measure of the uncertainty of a sample statistic such as the mean.[1]
**Difficulty level: 3**

**10 A** Sensitivity is a measure of a test's ability to identify true disease. Sensitivity is calculated by dividing the number of true-positive results by the total number of people with the disease (60/70). Specificity is a measure of a test's ability to correctly identify those without disease. Specificity is calculated by dividing the number of true negatives by the total number of people without disease (10/30).[1]
**Difficulty level: 3**

**11 A** Phase 1 trial: clinical pharmacology in normal volunteers assessing safety and dosage.
Phase 2 trial: preliminary small-scale studies.
Phase 3 trial: large-scale trials – application is made for a licence to sell the drug if it passes this test.
Phase 4 trial: post-marketing surveillance.[6]
**Difficulty level: 3**

**12 B** Parallax is a major issue when using an exophthalmometer and the devices have markers to help you line up the equipment correctly. Changing the base reading (distance between lateral orbital rims) can lead to variability from one measurement to the next. There can be a tendency to round off to the nearest 5 mm or 10 mm – this should be avoided. Use the same model of exophthalmometer when comparing readings as there may be subtle differences between the commonly used Oculus and Hertel exophthalmometers.[5]
**Difficulty level: 3**

**13 B** Primary prevention is designed to prevent disease; for example, by health education or controlling cardiac risk factors. Secondary prevention

aims to detect and treat the occurrence of disease before symptoms develop – most screening programmes fall into this category. Tertiary prevention is action to prevent sequelae once the disease is manifest.[6]
**Difficulty level: 2**

**14 A** Statistical tests are either parametric (i.e., they assume that the data were sampled from a particular form of distribution, such as a normal distribution) or non-parametric (they make no such assumption). In general, parametric tests are more powerful than non-parametric ones and so should be used if possible. Non-parametric tests look at the rank order of the values (which one is the smallest, which one comes next, and so on) and ignore the absolute differences between them. As you might imagine, statistical significance is more difficult to show with non-parametric tests. As height follows a normal distribution, a parametric test is appropriate.

Students often find it difficult to decide whether to use a paired or unpaired statistical test to analyse their data. If you measure something twice on each subject – for example, blood pressure measured when the subject is lying and when standing – you will probably be interested not just in the average difference of lying versus standing blood pressure in the entire sample, but in how much each individual's blood pressure changes with position. In this situation, you have what is called 'paired' data, because each measurement beforehand is paired with a measurement afterwards.

The two-sample (unpaired) T-test is a parametric test comparing two independent samples drawn from the same population. The Mann-Whitney U-test is the non-parametric equivalent of the two-sample (unpaired) T-test.[7]
**Difficulty level: 4**

**15 B** Pearson's correlation coefficient and Spearman's rank correlation coefficient assess the strength of the straight-line association between two continuous variables. Pearson's correlation coefficient is a parametric test and Spearman's rank correlation coefficient is the non-parametric equivalent.

Chi-squared and Fisher's exact test are non-parametric statistics testing the null hypothesis that the distribution of a discontinuous variable is the same in two (or more) independent samples. For example, these statistical tests could be used to assess whether acceptance into medical school is more likely if female.[7]
**Difficulty level: 4**

## References

1 Crawshaw J, Chambers J. *A Concise Course in A-Level Statistics.* 3rd ed. Cheltenham: Stanley Thornes; 1994. (**q1**) p. 125, (**q2**) p. 368, (**q8**) p. 508, (**q9**) pp. 443, 558, (**q10**) p. 224.

2 TL Jackson. *Moorfields Manual of Ophthalmology.* Philadelphia: Mosby Elsevier; 2008. (**q3**) p. 688, (**q4**) p. 689.

3 Batterbury M, Bowling B. *Ophthalmology – an illustrated colour text.* 1st ed. Edinburgh: Churchill Livingstone; 2002. (**q5**) p. 84.

4 The pyramid of evidence from different study designs. (Adapted from Medical Research Library of Brooklyn.) Available at: http://library.downstate.edu/EBM2/2100.htm (**q6**) (accessed 5 July 2011)

5 Madge S, Kersey J, Hawker M, *et al. Clinical Techniques in Ophthalmology.* Edinburgh: Churchill Livingstone; 2006. (**q7**) p. 277, (**q12**) p. 72.

6 Simon C, Everitt H, Birtwistle J, *et al. Oxford Handbook of General Practice.* Oxford: Oxford University Press; 2003. (**q11**) pp. 98–9, (**q13**) p. 80.

7 Greenhalgh T. How to read a paper: statistics for the non-statistician. I: Different types of data need different statistical tests. *BMJ.* 1997; **315**: 364–6 (**q14, q15**).

# 10. Epidemiology and biostatistics ICO answers

**16**   i. T       ii. F       iii. F       iv. T       v. T

The odds ratio of 'failure' in a test is the inverse of the odds ratio for 'success'. This symmetry of interpretation of the odds ratio is one of the reasons for its popularity. The same is not true of relative risks. It is important to consider the absolute risk and not just the relative risk in isolation – diseases that have low prevalence may require a very high relative risk to show a significant absolute risk increase, whereas highly prevalent diseases require only small increases in relative risk for significant numbers to be affected. In studies where the risk of disease is small, one would expect the relative risk and odds ratio to be close.[1]

**Difficulty level: 4**

**17**   i. T      ii. T      iii. T      iv. F      v. F

Sensitivity is a measure of a test's ability to identify true disease. Specificity is a measure of a test's ability to correctly identify those without disease. Positive predictive value equates to the number of true positives divided by the number who actually have the disease. Positive predictive value varies with disease prevalence.[1]

**Difficulty level: 2**

**18**   i. F      ii. F      iii. T      iv. T      v. T

Incidence is the number of new cases of disease per unit population per unit time. Prevalence measures the total number of cases of disease in a population at a particular point in time.[1]

**Difficulty level: 3**

**19**   i. F      ii. T      iii. F      iv. T      v. T

Driving must cease unless a patient is confirmed to meet the following visual field standard on Estermann binocular field testing: no visual field defect in the 120 degrees on the horizontal meridian measured using a target equivalent to the white Goldmann III4e settings. In addition, there should be no significant field defect encroaching within 20 degrees of fixation above or below the horizontal meridian. Significant field defect is defined as greater than three contiguous spots missed.[2]

**Difficulty level: 3**

**20**   i. T      ii. F      iii. T      iv. F      v. F

About 284 million people are visually impaired worldwide: 39 million are blind and 245 million have low vision. Eighty per cent of all visual impairment can be prevented, treated or cured. About 90% of the world's visually impaired people live in developing countries. Globally, uncorrected refractive errors are the main cause of visual impairment, while cataracts remain the leading cause of blindness. The number of people visually impaired from infectious diseases has greatly reduced in the last 20 years. Sixty-five per cent of visually impaired people are over 50 years of age, although this age group comprises only 20% of the world population. Top causes of visual impairment worldwide are refractive errors, cataracts and glaucoma.[3]

**Difficulty level: 4**

**21**   i. F      ii. F      iii. T      iv. T      v. F

Appointments can be missed due to patient or screening programme mistakes. Fail-safe mechanisms should be in place to at the very least inform the GP of non-attendance of the patient to screening. The screening interval should be shorter than the time taken for the disease to reach an untreatable stage. There should ideally be few false negatives and few false positives. If early treatment does not affect prognosis then it is questionable whether a screening programme is a good use of resources for that disease.[4]
   **Difficulty level: 1**

**22**   i. F      ii. F      iii. F      iv. T      v. T

The number needed to treat (NNT) is the inverse of the absolute risk reduction. The lower the NNT, the more effective the treatment. Thrombolysis in acute myocardial infarction has a NNT of approximately 8–20. The NNT depends on the baseline incidence of the disease. Take the following example regarding anti-hypertensive drugs to prevent vascular events, such as stroke or myocardial infarction. Sackett *et al.* (1997) showed that in patients with a diastolic blood pressure between 115 and 129 mmHg over 1.5 years, the NNT was 3. However, the use of the same drug in patients with a diastolic blood pressure between 90 and 109 mmHg with the same outcome over 5.5 years had an NNT of 128. The number needed to harm (NNH) is similar but represents the adverse effects from a therapy – the higher the number, the safer the treatment.[1]
   **Difficulty level: 4**

**23**   i. F      ii. T      iii. T      iv. T      v. T

A positive correlation does not in itself prove causality. There may be confounding factors that explain the positive correlation. Retrospective case-control studies are open to criticism for missing confounding factors. A well-designed appropriately powered prospective double-masked randomised control trial is the best way of eliminating confounding factors.[1]
   **Difficulty level: 2**

**24**   i. T      ii. F      iii. T      iv. T      v. T

A likelihood ratio > 1 indicates that the test result is associated with disease and < 1 that the test result is associated with absence of disease. A likelihood

ratio of 1 indicates the test is of no clinical value. However, it is not until the likelihood ratio is > 5 or < 0.2 that is becomes most useful.[1]
**Difficulty level: 3**

**25**  i. T    ii. T    iii. F    iv. T    v. F

The confidence interval (CI) helps to establish how certain we are that the sample data reflects the population. The narrower the CI, the more certain we can be the trial result is accurate. CI is normally expressed as 95% or approximately 2 standard deviations either side of the trial result. CI can only be applied to normally distributed parametric data.[1]
**Difficulty level: 3**

**26**  i. F    ii. F    iii. T    iv. T    v. F

The mean can be influenced by outliers and hence the median is a better measure of central tendency. Many distributions have more than one mode and are termed multimodal.[1]
**Difficulty level: 3**

**27**  i. T    ii. T    iii. T    iv. T    v. F

VISION 2020 is the global initiative for the elimination of avoidable blindness, a joint programme of the World Health Organization (WHO) and the International Agency for the Prevention of Blindness (IAPB) with an international membership of NGOs, professional associations, eye-care institutions and corporations. Diseases targeted include cataract, refractive error, trachoma, onchocerciasis, glaucoma, diabetic retinopathy and age-related macular degeneration.[5]
**Difficulty level: 3**

**28**  i. T    ii. T    iii. T    iv. T    v. T

It has been estimated that there are 1.4 million blind children in the world, 1 million of whom live in Asia and 300000 in Africa. Owing to demographic differences, the number of children who are blind per 10 million population varies from approximately 600 in affluent countries to approximately 6000 in very poor communities. About 40% of the causes of childhood blindness are preventable or treatable. The main causes of blindness in children change over time. As a consequence of child survival programmes (for example, integrated management of childhood illness), corneal scarring due to measles and vitamin A deficiency is declining in many developing countries, so that the proportion due to cataract is increasing. Retinopathy of prematurity is emerging as an important cause in the middle-income countries of Latin America and Eastern Europe and is likely to become an important cause in Asia over the next decade. The prevalence of refractive errors, particularly myopia, is increasing in school-age children, especially in Southeast Asia.[6]

**Difficulty level: 3**

**29**  i.  T   ii.  F   iii.  F   iv.  F   v.  F

In single-masked trials the patient does not know which intervention they are having. In double-masked trials investigators and those analysing data are also unaware which treatment the patient is having. Masking reduces selection and interpretation bias. Masking is preferred to the term blinding when dealing with the field of ophthalmology. Publication bias is the publication of trials, by researchers, pharmaceutical companies and journals that are positive rather than negative.[1]

**Difficulty level: 3**

**30**  i.  T   ii.  T   iii.  T   iv.  F   v.  F

Pearsons correlation coefficient should be used for normally distributed data. It is a parametric test. Values range between −1 (negative correlation) and +1 (positive correlation), with 0 indicating no correlation. Spearman's rank correlation coefficient ranks the data points for variables x and y and makes no assumptions about the underlying distribution of the data – it is a non-parametric test.[1]

**Difficulty level: 3**

## References

1 Campbell MJ, Machin D, Walters SJ. *Medical Statistics*. 4th ed. London: John Wiley & Sons; 2007. **(q16)** pp. 20–1, **(q17)** pp. 49–51, **(q18)** pp. 219–20, **(q22)** p. 259, **(q23)** pp. 237–8, **(q24)** p. 54, **(q25)** p. 111, **(q26)** p. 28, **(q29)** p. 248, **(q30)** p. 156.

2 Jackson TL. *Moorfields Manual of Ophthalmology*. Philadelphia: Mosby Elsevier; 2008. **(q19)** p. 688.

3 www.vision2020.org/main.cfm?type=FACTS **(q20)** (accessed 5 July 2011)

4 Simon C, Everitt H, Birtwistle J, *et al. Oxford Handbook of General Practice.* 1st ed. Oxford: Oxford University Press; 2002. (**q21**) pp. 80–1.

5 www.vision2020.org/main.cfm?type=WHATVISION2020 (**q27**) (accessed 5 July 2011)

6 www.vision2020.org/main.cfm?type=WIBCHILDHOOD (**q28**) (accessed 5 July 2011)

# 11. Clinical genetics FRCOphth answers

**1  B**  A chromosome is made up of double-stranded DNA wrapped around histone proteins, and this DNA-protein complex is called chromatin. Each chromosome comprises of two sister chromatids, which are joined at the centromere. It is the centromere that attaches to the spindle fibres in cell division before the sister chromatids separate.[1]
**Difficulty level: 2**

**2  D**  In transcription, an RNA copy is made from the DNA sequence of the relevant gene. It begins when a large complex of proteins assembles at a particular site of the DNA, usually the promoter sequence. The DNA contains exons (coding sequences) and introns (non-coding sequences), which are both transcribed. Subsequently the introns are spliced out by the spliceosome, resulting in messenger RNA. Ribosomes are involved in translation of messenger RNA into protein.[1]
**Difficulty level: 2**

**3  C**  Penetrance is the proportion of people with a particular genotype that show characteristics of the condition or phenotype associated with it. For example, if a person possessed the genotype associated with an autosomal dominant condition but was asymptomatic, this is non-penetrance.

Variable expressivity is seen in genetic conditions with multiple features (such as neurofibromatosis), when those affected show only some of the associated features.

Anticipation is the tendency for a disease to become more severe, frequent or have earlier onset with successive generations. It is often seen in disorders involving expansion of a nucleotide repeat such as Huntington's disease.

Mosaicism occurs when an organism consists of two or more genetically different cell lines. It arises since mutations may occur in a cell at any time, and the descendants of only that cell will contain the mutation. It is of no significance unless the mutation occurs in a germ line cell.[1]
**Difficulty level: 3**

4  **A**  Polymorphisms in the complement factor H gene have been shown to be associated with age-related macular degeneration. *BEST1* mutations are associated with Best macular dystrophy, *ABCA4* gene mutations with Stargardt disease and *RPE65* with Leber's congenital amaurosis. Gene therapy replacement of *RPE65* is currently in the clinical trial phase.[2,3]
**Difficulty level: 3**

5  **A**  Translocated chromosomes have segments derived from more than one chromosome. If the translocation is balanced (i.e., no genetic material is added or deleted), the patient may be asymptomatic provided that the break is not through a gene or a regulatory sequence. If a translocation results in deletion or addition of genetic material, this is more likely to be pathological.[1]
**Difficulty level: 2**

6  **B**  In aneuploid cells, an incorrect number of chromosomes are present. In Turner's syndrome only one sex chromosome is present (XO). Other examples are Down's syndrome (trisomy 21), Edwards' syndrome (trisomy 18) and Patau syndrome (trisomy 13). In Kleinfelter syndrome there is an extra X chromosome (XXY).

Myotonic dystrophy, Marfan's syndrome and albinism are all gene disorders rather than chromosomal disorders.[1]
**Difficulty level: 3**

7  **B**  In X-linked disorders such as X-linked retinitis pigmentosa, the defective gene is on the X chromosome. Therefore males are affected if they possess this X chromosome, but females are carriers since they also possess a normal X chromosome. Father-to-son transmission is not seen. Affected individuals may have affected maternal uncles, and subsequent brothers have a 1 in 2 risk of being affected. Sisters have a 1 in 2 risk of being carriers.[1]
**Difficulty level: 3**

**8  D**  Mitochondrial disorders arise due to dysfunction of the mitochondrial respiratory chain. Some disorders such as Leber's hereditary optic neuropathy generally affect the eye only, whereas others such as Kearns-Sayre syndrome have multiple features including pigmentary retinopathy, heart block, cerebellar ataxia and myopathy. In chronic progressive external ophthalmoplegia, along with ophthalmoplegia there is bilateral ptosis and sometimes mild proximal myopathy.

Neurofibromatosis type 2 is inherited in an autosomal dominant pattern.[4]

**Difficulty level: 3**

**9  A**  Northern blotting is used to detect RNA, Southern blotting to detect DNA and Western blotting to detect protein. Eastern blotting does not exist. In Southern blotting, for example, once the DNA has been isolated from a tissue, gel electrophoresis is used to separate the DNA sample into its constituent components, as longer segments of DNA run more slowly through the gel than shorter sections. The gel is then transferred to a membrane and the target DNA sequence is identified using a hybridisation probe. A similar principle applies to Northern and Western blotting.[5]

**Difficulty level: 3**

**10  A**  The polymerase chain reaction (PCR) is a technique widely used in molecular biology to amplify DNA. The important constituents include a DNA template, a DNA polymerase, two primers, buffer solution and deoxynucleoside triphosphates – the building blocks from which the DNA polymerase synthesizes a new DNA strand.

A high temperature is used to denature DNA and separate the two complementary strands. Primers, designed to be complementary to short sections of each of the forward and reverse single strands, are included in the PCR mixture. By lowering the temperature, the primers anneal to the single-stranded DNA. From the site where the primers have bound, DNA polymerase then synthesises a new strand of complementary DNA. As PCR progresses, the DNA generated is itself used as a template for replication and a chain reaction is set up, in which the DNA template is exponentially amplified.[6]

**Difficulty level: 3**

**11  C**  The stages of mitosis are as follows:

Prophase: chromatin condenses to form chromosomes.

Metaphase: nuclear membrane disappears and chromosomes convene along the equatorial plate.

Anaphase: the proteins that bind sister chromatids together are cleaved, allowing them to separate and they move apart to opposite ends of the cell.

Telophase: a new nuclear envelope forms around the separated sister chromosomes, and the chromosomes unfold back into chromatin.[1]
**Difficulty level: 4**

**12 C** The ribosome is the cellular structure in which proteins are synthesised. Translation is the process in which a polypeptide chain is formed from messenger RNA (*not* transcription). Ribosomes are bound to the rough endoplasmic reticulum as well as floating freely in the cytoplasm. They are comprised of two subunits – a small subunit to which messenger RNA and transfer RNA bringing amino acids attach, and a large subunit which provides enzymes that link amino acids to form a peptide.[7]
**Difficulty level: 3**

**13 B** Genetic drift is a change in gene frequency between generations. It arises due to chance differences between the gene frequency in one generation and the genes passed on to their gametes. Gene flow may be defined as the transfer of alleles from one population to another. Mutations are changes to the nucleotide sequence of the genetic material of an organism. Natural selection is the process whereby favourable heritable traits become more common in successive generations, with unfavourable traits becoming less common.[1]
**Difficulty level: 3**

**14 D** Gene therapy involves the modification of genetic material in the cells of an organism in order to treat disease. Viral vectors are used most commonly for the delivery of genetic material to the cells: adeno-associated virus and lentiviruses such as human immunodeficiency virus 1 and feline immunodeficiency virus have been successfully used for this purpose in animal models. In the human clinical trial to treat patients with Leber's congenital amaurosis, adeno-associated viruses were used. Rhinovirus is not used for the purpose of gene therapy.[8]
**Difficulty level: 4**

**15 A** Edwards' syndrome is trisomy of chromosome 18. Those with Turner's syndrome have only one sex chromosome (XO). Vogt-Koyanagi-Harada syndrome is an autoimmune disease with inflammation targeted at melanocytes, such as in the uveal tract. It is associated with HLA-DR1 and HLA-DR4. Stickler's syndrome is a disorder of collagen, with over 60% of patients having a mutation in the *COL2A1* gene. It is inherited in an autosomal dominant manner with variable expressivity. It results in high myopia and retinal detachment.[9]

**Difficulty level: 4**

## References

1 Read A, Donnai D. *New Clinical Genetics*. 1st ed. Banbury: Scion Publishing; 2007. **(q1)** pp. 33–5, **(q2)** pp. 60–1, **(q3)** pp. 16–21, **(q5)** p. 47, **(q6)** p. 32, **(q7)** p. 14, **(q11)** p. 35, **(q13)** p. 405.

2 Klein RJ, Zeiss C, Chew EY, *et al.* Complement factor H polymorphism in age-related macular degeneration. *Science.* 2005; **308**(5720): 385–9 **(q4)**.

3 Bainbridge JW, Smith AJ, Barker SS, *et al.* Effect of gene therapy on visual function in Leber's congenital amaurosis. *N Engl J Med.* 2008; **358**(21): 2231–9 **(q4)**.

4 Chinnery PF. Mitochondrial Disorders Overview. Available at: www.ncbi.nlm.nih.gov/books/NBK1224 **(q8)** (accessed 5 July 2011)

5 Southern EM. Detection of specific sequences among DNA fragments separated by gel electrophoresis. *J Mol Biol.* 1975; **98**: 503–17 **(q9)**.

6 Wilson K, Walker J. *Principles and Techniques of Biochemistry and Molecular Biology.* 7th ed. Cambridge: Cambridge University Press; 2010. **(q10)** pp. 179–85.

7 Guyton A, Hall J. *Textbook of Medical Physiology.* 11th ed. Philadelphia: Saunders Elsevier; 2006. **(q12)** p. 33.

8 Bainbridge JW, Tan MH, Ali RR. Gene therapy progress and prospects: the eye. *Gene Ther.* 2006; **13**(16): 1191–7 **(q14)**.

9 Kanski JJ. *Clinical Ophthalmology – a systematic approach.* 6th ed. Edinburgh: Butterworth Heinemann Elsevier; 2007. **(q15)** pp. 880, 888.

# 11. Clinical genetics ICO answers

**16**  i. F    ii. T    iii. T    iv. T    v. F

Linkage analysis depends on the behaviour of chromosomes at meiosis. Non-homologous chromosomes, chromosomes that are not from the same pair, independently assort to the resultant gametes in meiosis. Chromosomes from the same pair, once they are aligned in meiosis, can undergo crossing over with an allele being passed from one chromosome to its paired chromosome.

In gene mapping, it is assumed that two loci on the same chromosome will be passed on together unless crossing over occurs. Crossover is more likely if the loci are further apart than if they are close together. Loci that undergo crossing over in 1% of cases are defined as being 1 centimorgan apart.

The Lod score is a statistical measure that indicates how significant the chance of linkage is. Patients with aneuploidy have an incorrect number of chromosomes, therefore karyotyping would be the appropriate test in these patients.[1]

**Difficulty level: 4**

**17**   i. T       ii. T       iii. F       iv. T       v. F

Retinoblastoma is the most common primary intraocular malignancy of childhood. Approximately 40% of cases are heritable and 60% non-heritable. It arises due to a mutation in the retinoblastoma tumour suppressor gene (*RB1*) on chromosome 13. Knudson's two-hit hypothesis postulates that in heritable retinoblastoma, mutation in one allele is inherited and present in all body cells. A sporadic further event then affects the second allele and the cell undergoes malignant transformation. These children may develop bilateral retinoblastomas and also pinealomas, so are said to have trilateral disease. The mutations in both alleles in non-heritable disease are sporadic, and the children have unilateral disease.[2]

**Difficulty level: 3**

**18**   i. T       ii. F       iii. T       iv. F       v. T

In DNA replication, initially the double stranded DNA helix is unwound and separated into single strands – this is catalysed by a DNA helicase (or can also be done in vitro by high temperatures). The single-stranded DNA acts as a template. DNA polymerase assists with DNA replication by catalysing the step-wise addition of nucleotides to a primer strand that is paired to the DNA template strand. DNA polymerase requires magnesium as a co-factor. It is DNA ligase that joins the ends of *double-stranded* DNA together with a covalent bond to make a continuous DNA strand.[3]

**Difficulty level: 4**

**19**   i. F       ii. F       iii. T       iv. T       v. F

The bestrophin-1 protein encoded by the *BEST1* gene is a chloride channel, predominantly expressed in the retinal pigment epithelium. Mutations in *BEST1* may cause:

a) vitelliform macular dystrophy (Best disease), inherited in an autosomal dominant pattern
b) adult-onset macular vitelliform dystrophy – 25% of cases are due to mutations in *BEST1*; these may be sporadic or inherited in an autosomal dominant pattern
c) autosomal recessive bestrophinopathy
d) autosomal dominant vitreoretinochoroidopathy (ADVIRC). Mutations in *BEST1* cause an abnormal EOG (except in some patients with adult-onset vitelliform dystrophy in which it can be normal).[4]
**Difficulty level: 5**

**20** i. F ii. F iii. T iv. F v. T

A DNA strand consists of nucleotide units linked by phosphate bonds. A nucleotide consists of a pentose sugar, phosphate group and a base. DNA can form a double-stranded structure due to the formation of hydrogen bonds between complementary base pairs on two DNA strands. Only two base pairings may occur: guanine to cytosine and also adenine and thymine. The double-stranded DNA then forms a helical structure.[5]
**Difficulty level: 3**

**21** i. F ii. T iii. T iv. F v. F

Meiosis is a specialised form of cell division in by which gametes are formed in eukaryotic cells only. The resultant gametes are all genetically unique. Meiosis is preceded by the S phase of the cell cycle (in which there is DNA replication). During prophase I, the chromosomes condense and pair and there is recombination of genetic material between homologous chromosomes. At the end of meiosis I, each daughter cell has 23 chromosomes. In meiosis II the sister chromatids separate, in a similar way to mitosis.[1]
**Difficulty level: 3**

**22** i. F ii. F iii. F iv. T v. T

In X-linked inheritance, males carrying the disease gene are affected and women are carriers. In this case the mother (X'X) and father (XY) will have children with the following genotypes: X'X, X'Y, XX, XY. Therefore half the sons are affected, half the daughters are carriers. Overall one-quarter of children are affected by the disease.[1]
**Difficulty level: 3**

**23**   i. F     ii. T     iii. F     iv. F     v. F

The condition is autosomal dominant, and assuming the parents are hetero-zygotes with genotype P'P and Q'Q, the children will have genotypes P'Q', P'Q, PQ' and PQ. Therefore, three-quarters will be affected. In an autosomal dominant condition, there is no carrier state and no sex bias.[1]
   **Difficulty level: 3**

**24**   i. F     ii. F     iii. T     iv. F     v. F

Restriction enzyme digestion can be used in the diagnosis of inherited dis-eases, in which the mutation affects the restriction site. Southern blotting can be used to detect certain DNA sequences, but both of the above techniques require large amounts of DNA so are not suitable to be done from viral swabs. In PCR, primers specific to the viral DNA sequence can be used to identify and amplify this DNA relatively quickly. Reverse transcriptase PCR uses RNA as a substrate so is used if an RNA virus is suspected, or to assess which genes are being expressed in a cell. Gram staining identifies bacteria.[6]
   **Difficulty level: 2**

**25**   i. T     ii. F     iii. F     iv. T     v. F

In nonsense mutations, one nucleotide is replaced by another which changes a codon to a stop codon. The ribosome would theoretically then detach and protein synthesis be terminated at this point. However, the majority of mRNA containing a premature stop codon undergoes nonsense-mediated decay. Thus no protein is formed and the result of the nonsense mutation may be the same as a complete gene deletion.

   A missense mutation involves one nucleotide being replaced by another causing a codon change, resulting in one amino acid being replaced with another. A frame shift only occurs when nucleotides are added or deleted in multiples of greater or less than three. This changes the downstream reading of the DNA beyond this point.[1]
   **Difficulty level: 4**

**26**   i. T     ii. F     iii. F     iv. F     v. T

Transcription is initiated by the binding of transcription factors to DNA within the promoter sequence. An example of a site that a general transcrip-tion factor binds to is the TATA box (a sequence of T and A nucleotides within the promoter). RNA polymerase II then assembles at the promoter site, initi-ating transcription. The mRNA that is produced undergoes splicing to remove introns. DNA polymerase is required in DNA replication.[3]

**Difficulty level: 4**

**27**    i. T      ii. T      iii. F      iv. T      v. F

Adoption studies aim to investigate the effects of genes versus family envir-onment. Twin studies compare monozygotic and dizygotic twins: a higher concordance of a phenotype in monozygotic twins gives evidence for genetic factors. Association studies look at the relationship between alleles and pheno-types to examine whether a particular marker allele is associated with a disease phenotype.

Karyotyping is an examination of chromosomes. Restriction enzyme digestion may identify specific gene defects since the mutation may alter the restriction site.[1]

**Difficulty level: 3**

**28**    i. F      ii. T      iii. F      iv. T      v. F

There is no connection between the frequency of an allele and whether it causes a dominant or recessive phenotype. Therefore, an allele that causes a dominant phenotype is not necessarily more common. Heterozygote advan-tage may lead to a recessive allele being more common in a population, such as the protective advantage of being a sickle-cell heterozygote with respect to malaria.

Gene frequency is a balance between mutations and natural selection. The latter acts to reduce the presence of a dominant mutation in the population, and also a recessive mutation when it is in the homozygous form (i.e. it is manifest).

The Hardy-Weinberg distribution describes the relationship between genotype frequencies and gene frequencies.[1]

**Difficulty level: 3**

**29**    i. F      ii. T      iii. F      iv. T      v. F

Cloning a gene involves its insertion into a vector such as a plasmid. This is an often circular segment of DNA that can replicate independently of the chromosomal DNA. In order to insert a gene, the plasmid needs to be cut. This is done with restriction endonucleases, which are enzymes that cut DNA of a specific sequence. The ends of the gene are also cut with the enzyme so the ends of the plasmid and gene are complementary. The two are then joined by DNA ligase.[1]

**Difficulty level: 3**

**30**   i.  F        ii.  F        iii.  F        iv.  T        v.  F

Most corneal dystrophies are inherited in an autosomal dominant manner or are sporadic. Macular dystrophy, lattice dystrophy type 3 and congenital hereditary endothelial dystrophy type 2 are among the few that are inherited in an autosomal recessive manner.[2]

**Difficulty level: 4**

## References

1  Read A, Donnai D. *New Clinical Genetics*. 1st ed. Banbury: Scion Publishing; 2007. (**q16**) p. 232, (**q21**) pp. 35–7, (**q22, q23**) p. 14, (**q25**) pp. 144–6, (**q27**) pp. 333–41, (**q28**) pp. 262–4, (**q29**) p. 92.
2  Kanski JJ. *Clinical Ophthalmology – a systematic approach*. 6th ed. Edinburgh: Butterworth Heinemann Elsevier; 2007. (**q17**) pp. 542–5, (**q30**) pp. 290–302.
3  Alberts B, Johnson A, Lewis J, *et al. Molecular Biology of the Cell*. 4th ed. New York: Garland Science; 2002. (**q 18**) Chapter 5, (**q26**) Chapter 6.
4  Camiel JF, Boona B, Kleveringa J, *et al*. The spectrum of ocular phenotypes caused by mutations in the *BEST1* gene. *Prog Retin Eye Res*. 2009; **28**(3): 187–205 (**q19**).
5  Colledge NR, Walker BR, Ralston SH. *Davidson's Principles and Practice of Medicine*. 21st ed. Edinburgh: Churchill Livingstone Elsevier; 2010. (**q20**) pp. 40–1.
6  Wilson K, Walker J. *Principles and Techniques of Biochemistry and Molecular Biology*. 7th ed. Cambridge: Cambridge University Press; 2010. (**q24**) pp. 172, 185.

# 12.  Patient investigation FRCOphth answers

**1**   **C**   Fluorescein causes temporary discoloration of skin and urine. Mild side effects include nausea, vomiting, flushing of skin and itching. Serious but rare problems include syncope, laryngeal oedema and anaphylactic shock. Therefore, it is important to have appropriate life-support measures

in place. Vortex keratopathy (corneal verticillata) are whorl-like corneal epithelial deposits. The most common causes are amiodarone- and chloroquine-derived drugs. They are not associated with fluorescein.[1]
**Difficulty level: 1**

2   **B**   The choroidal (pre-arterial) phase occurs 8–12 seconds after dye injection and is characterised by patchy filling of the choroid due to leakage of free fluorescein through the fenestrated choriocapillaris. The rate and site of fluorescein injection, age of the patient and cardiovascular status can affect the time it takes for fluorescein to reach the ocular circulation.[1]
**Difficulty level: 3**

3   **C**   If an intraocular or intraorbital metallic foreign body is suspected, MRI scanning is contraindicated. Electronically, magnetically and mechanically activated implants such as cardiac pacemakers, ferromagnetic or electronically operated stapedial implants and aneurysm clips are contraindications to MRI scanning.[1]
**Difficulty level: 2**

4   **C**   A-scan ultrasonography is performed with a single ultrasound source. It produces a one-dimensional time-amplitude evaluation in the form of vertical spikes along a baseline. The height of the spikes is proportional to the strength of the echo. The distance between individual spikes can be precisely measured.[1]
**Difficulty level: 3**

5   **B**   OCT is analogous to B-scan ultrasonography but uses light instead of sound waves. The Heidelberg Retina Tomograph (HRT) is a scanning laser ophthalmoscope that can interpret differences in the profile of the optic nerve head and peripapillary nerve fibre layer to produce a 3D topographical map. GDx VCC measures the change in polarisation caused by the birefringence of nerve fibre layer axons.[1]
**Difficulty level: 3**

6   **B**   A is a definition of total deviation. C is a definition of global indices. D is a definition of differential light sensitivity. Media opacities and miosis are common reasons for generalised depressions in the visual field that can be adjusted for with the pattern deviation.[1]
**Difficulty level: 3**

**7  B**   Each letter is composed of five elements. Each element subtends 1 minute of arc when the 6/6 letter is viewed at 6 metres.[1]
**Difficulty level: 2**

**8  C**   ESR is often very high with levels of > 60 mm/hour. Elevated CRP and thrombocytosis are also associated with temporal arteritis. Rarely, biopsy-proven temporal arteritis can occur in the presence of normal ESR and CRP. Neither elevated ESR, CRP nor platelet count is specific to temporal arteritis.[1]
**Difficulty level: 2**

**9  B**   Gram staining differentiates bacterial species into Gram-positive and Gram-negative based on the ability of the crystal violet dye to penetrate the cell wall.[1]
**Difficulty level: 3**

**10  C**   Bone mineral density (BMD) testing generally correlates with bone strength and its ability to bear weight. The BMD is measured with a dual energy X-ray absorptiometry test (referred to as a DEXA scan). By measuring BMD, it is possible to predict fracture risk. Stem 10A is the normal range for BMD. Stem 10B is the definition for osteopaenia.[2]
**Difficulty level: 3**

**11  C**   Direct illumination with diffuse light allows visualisation of a cross section of the cornea. Retroillumination uses light reflected from the iris to illuminate the cornea, and allows detection of subtle endothelial changes. Scleral scatter involves decentration of the slit lamp laterally so that the light is incident on the limbus with the microscope focused centrally. With scleral scatter, light is then transmitted within the cornea by total internal reflection highlighting stromal lesions.[1]
**Difficulty level: 3**

**12  B**   The Hess chart plots the dissociated ocular position as a function of the extraocular muscles. Each square on the Hess Chart equals 5 degrees of arc. Hess charts enable differentiation of paretic strabismus caused by neurological pathology from restrictive myopathy. Hess charts are also useful for differentiating recent-onset from long-standing deficits.[1]
**Difficulty level: 3**

**13  C**   The SRK I and SRK II formulae are obsolete and should no longer be used. Which modern IOL calculation formula (SRK/T, Holladay I & II, Haigis and Hoffer Q) gives the best results has been subject to debate.

All modern formulae perform well in the normal axial length range but the Haigis and Hoffer Q may be slightly better for short axial lengths (< 22 mm).[3]
**Difficulty level: 3**

**14 C** Slit-lamp examination can demonstrate corneal thinning, Vogt striae and Fleischer rings. Retinoscopy shows an irregular scissor reflex in more advanced keratoconus. Corneal topography shows irregular astigmatism and is the most sensitive method of detecting early keratoconus and in monitoring progression.[1]
**Difficulty level: 2**

**15 B** The Ziehl–Neelsen test is useful for the staining of *Mycobacterium* and *Nocardia*, which it stains bright red. Because of its lipid-rich cell wall, *Mycobacterium tuberculosis* does not stain well with Gram staining.[4]
**Difficulty level: 2**

## References

1 Kanski JJ, *Clinical Ophthalmology*. 6th ed. Edinburgh: Butterworth Heinmann, Elsevier; 2007. (**q1**) pp. 37, 839, (**q2**) pp. 37–9, (**q3**) p. 55, (**q4**) p. 44, (**q5**) pp. 47–52, (**q6**) p. 29, (**q7**) p. 15, (**q8**) p. 878, (**q9, q11**) p. 256, (**q12**) pp. 761–2, (**q14**) p. 288.

2 www.medicinenet.com/bone_density_scan (**q10**) (accessed 5 July 2011)

3 Maclaren RE, Natkunarajah M, Riaz Y, *et al.* Biometry and formula accuracy with intraocular lenses used for cataract surgery in extreme hyperopia. *Am J Ophthalmol.* 2007; **143**: 920–31 (**q13**).

4 Forrester J, Dick A, McMenamin A, *et al. The Eye: basic sciences in practice*. 2nd ed. Philadelphia: Saunders Elsevier; 2007. (**q15**) p. 364.

# 12. Patient investigation ICO answers

**16**   i. T       ii. T       iii. T       iv. F       v. F

In corneal topography, steep curvatures are represented by warm colours and flat curvatures by cold colours. An absolute scale should always be used to facilitate comparison over time and between patients. Relative (normalised) scales are not fixed and colours vary.[1]
   **Difficulty level: 3**

**17**   i. T       ii. T       iii. T       iv. T       v. T

ICG fluoresces in the infrared range of wavelengths. Normal RPE pigments do not block the infrared radiation; thus, by using a specially adapted camera to capture the emitted infrared rays, information can be obtained about the choroidal circulation, which might not be available from fluorescein angiography.[1]
   **Difficulty level: 3**

**18**   i. F       ii. T       iii. T       iv. T       v. F

An advantage of MRI is that it does not expose the patient to ionising radiation. MRI is poor at detecting bone and it therefore appears black. Fat-suppression techniques attempt to overcome the problem of obscuration of orbital contents by the bright signal from orbital fat in $T_1$-weighted images. Therefore, it is important to inform the radiographer which structures you are interested in imaging. Gadolinium is used to enhance $T_1$-weighted images – it is not visible on $T_2$-weighted images.[1]
   **Difficulty level: 3**

**19**   i. F       ii. T       iii. F       iv. T       v. T

CT scanning is widely available, easy to perform, relatively inexpensive, takes only a few minutes to perform and is generally well tolerated by claustrophobic patients. It can be used when MRI is contraindicated, such as in patients with suspected intraocular ferrous foreign bodies. MRI is preferable to CT when imaging soft tissue injuries.[1]
   **Difficulty level: 2**

**20**   i. T   ii. T   iii. T   iv. F   v. T

OCT requires the media to be clear enough to detect backscatter of light from the retinal layers. Fourier-domain scanners show greater detail and shorter acquisition time than time-domain scanners. Therefore, Fourier-domain scanners have dramatically reduced motion artefact.[2]

**Difficulty level: 5**

**21**   i. T   ii. F   iii. F   iv. T   v. T

The Humphrey perimeter has a range of static perimetry strategies (e.g. 30-1, 24-2). The number before the dash indicates the area of field tested in degrees from fixation. The 24-degree strategy tests 54 points. The number after the dash describes the pattern of points presented to the patient. The SITA program does not use the conventional staircase method to establish thresholds, thereby allowing the test to be faster.[1]

**Difficulty level: 3**

**22**   i. F   ii. T   iii. F   iv. F   v. T

Cone flicker is used to isolate cones by using a flickering light stimulus at a frequency of 30 Hz to which rods cannot respond. Cone responses can be elicited in normal eyes up to 50 Hz, after which point individual responses are no longer recordable (critical flicker fusion). Rod responses are elicited with a very dim flash of white light or a blue light resulting in a large b-wave and a small or non-recordable a-wave.[1]

**Difficulty level: 4**

**23**   i. T   ii. F   iii. F   iv. F   v. T

The EOG measures the standing potential between the electrically positive cornea and the electrically negative retina/RPE complex. It reflects the activity of the RPE and photoreceptors. There is much variation in EOG absolute amplitudes in normal subjects. Therefore, a ratio of the light peak to the dark trough is used to determine the Arden ratio. The normal Arden ratio is 1.85.[1]

**Difficulty level: 3**

**24**   i. T        ii. T        iii. T        iv. F        v. T

In albinism, the optic chiasm has more crossed nerve fibres than normal and this can be demonstrated on VEP studies.[1]
   **Difficulty level: 3**


**25**   i. F        ii. T        iii. T        iv. F        v. T

In primary hypothyroidism, the thyroid hormone levels are reduced and the TSH levels are elevated. Systemically ill patients can have apparently low thyroid hormone levels and TSH levels – the 'sick euthyroid' syndrome. Drugs such as phenytoin can cause altered binding of thyroid hormones to thyroxine-binding globulin and therefore thyroid function tests should be interpreted with caution in this situation. In Graves' disease, thyroid eye disease can develop independent of the patient's thyroid status.[3]
   **Difficulty level: 3**


**26**   i. T        ii. T        iii. F        iv. T        v. T

Increased expiration of carbon dioxide leads to respiratory alkalosis. Retention of carbon dioxide, for example due to weakness of thoracic muscles in Guillain-Barré syndrome, causes respiratory acidosis. Diabetic ketoacidosis causes a metabolic acidosis. Loss of gastric fluid rich in acid during vomiting results in a metabolic alkalosis. Acetazolamide causes increased renal bicarbonate loss leading to a metabolic acidosis.[3]
   **Difficulty level: 4**


**27**   i. F        ii. T        iii. F        iv. F        v. F

Proteinuria is one of the commonest signs of renal disease. Normal individuals excrete about 40 mg of albumin per day. Most urine dipstick reagents detect protein levels at a concentration of 100 mg/L (approx 150 mg of albumin a day). An increase in albumin levels between these two levels is termed micro-albuminuria – an early indicator of glomerular disease. Exercise, adopting an upright position and pyrexia can increase urinary protein output. Renal glycosuria is uncommon, so that a positive test for glucose always requires exclusion of diabetes mellitus. Menstruation in females can account for blood in the urine.[3]
   **Difficulty level: 3**

**28**  i. T  ii. F  iii. T  iv. T  v. F

MHC is a cluster of genes located on the short arm of chromosome 6 coding HLA antigens. HLA molecules are distributed throughout the body tissues and it is through differences in HLA that cells are classified as self or non-self. Class 1 HLA antigens (HLA-A, B and C) are expressed on all cell types except erythrocytes and trophoblasts. Class 2 HLA antigens (HLA-D, -DR and D-related) are expressed on antigen presenting cells and activated T-cells.[3]

**Difficulty level: 4**


**29**  i. T  ii. T  iii. F  iv. F  v. T

It is important during the cover/uncover test not to dissociate the eyes as this will uncover a latent component of the squint which you are not attempting to measure. In the alternate cover test, dissociation of the eyes allows the latent component also to be measured. The cover test can be used for horizontal and vertical deviations.[4]

**Difficulty level: 3**


**30**  i. T  ii. F  iii. F  iv. T  v. F

Necrotic cardiac tissue releases several enzymes and proteins into the serum. CK is produced by damaged skeletal muscle and brain as well as cardiac tissue. LDH is a non-tissue-specific enzyme. Its main use is in late detection (up to 10 days) of MI. Troponin T and I are cardiac selective. They are released from 2 to 4 hours following the MI and remain elevated for up to 7 days.[3]

**Difficulty level: 3**


## References

1 Kanski JJ. *Clinical Ophthalmology – a systematic approach.* 6th ed. Edinburgh: Butterworth Heinemann Elsevier; 2007. (**q16**) pp. 33–4, (**q17**) p. 42, (**q18**) p. 55, (**q19**) p. 52, (**q21**) pp. 27–9, (**q22**) p. 22, (**q23**) p. 23, (**q24**) pp. 24, 669.

2 Regillo CD, editor. *Fundamentals and Principles of Ophthalmology Part XII: retina and vitreous.* San Francisco: American Academy of Ophthalmology Basic and Clinical Science Course 2010–2011. (**q20**) p. 27.

3 Kumar P, Clark M. *Clinical Medicine.* 5th ed. Edinburgh: WB Saunders; 2002. (**q25**) pp. 1036–40, (**q26**) pp. 689–97, (**q27**) p. 595, (**q28**) p. 205, (**q30**) p. 777.

4 Madge S, Kersey J, Hawker M, *et al. Clinical Techniques in Ophthalmology.* Edinburgh: Churchill Livingstone; 2006. pp. 113–16 (**q29**).

# Index

*Please note: Page numbers are given in the following format Q/A where Q = 'Question' and A = 'Answer'*

#0231 - 150317 - C0 - 246/174/19 - PB - 9781846195464